Occupational Therapy Evidence in Practice for Mental Health

Occupational Therapy Evidence in Practice for Mental Health

Edited by

C. Long
and
J. Cronin-Davis

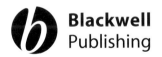

Blackwell
Publishing

Editorial offices:
Blackwell Publishing Ltd, 9600 Garsington Road, Oxford OX4 2DQ, UK
Tel: +44 (0)1865 776868
Blackwell Publishing Inc., 350 Main Street, Malden, MA 02148–5020, USA
Tel: +1 781 388 8250
Blackwell Publishing Asia Pty Ltd, 550 Swanston Street, Carlton, Victoria 3053, Australia
Tel: +61 (0)3 8359 1011

First published 2006 by Blackwell Publishing Ltd

ISBN-13: 978-1-4051-4666-1
ISBN-10: 1-4051-4666-4

Library of Congress Cataloging-in-Publication Data
Occupational therapy evidence in practice for mental health / edited by C. Long and
    J. Cronin-Davis.
        p. ; cm.
    Includes bibliographical references and index.
    ISBN-13: 978-1-4051-4666-1 (pbk. : alk. paper)
    ISBN-10: 1-4051-4666-4 (pbk. : alk. paper)
    1. Mentally ill–Rehabilitation.   2. Occupational therapy   I. Long, C. (Cathy)   II. Cronin-Davis, J. (Jane)
    [DNLM: 1. Mental Disorders–therapy.   2. Occupational Therapy–methods.   3. Evidence-Based Medicine. WM 450.5.O2 O146 2006]
    RC439.5.O23 2006
    616.89′165–dc22
    2006010837

A catalogue record for this title is available from the British Library
Set in 10 on 12.5 pt Palatino
by SNP Best-set Typesetter Ltd., Hong Kong
Printed and bound in India
by Replika Press Put Ltd, Kundli

The publisher's policy is to use permanent paper from mills that operate a sustainable forestry policy, and which has been manufactured from pulp processed using acid-free and elementary chlorine-free practices. Furthermore, the publisher ensures that the text paper and cover board used have met acceptable environmental accreditation standards.

For further information on Blackwell Publishing, visit our website:
www.blackwellpublishing.com

Contents

Preface

Editing this book has for us been an interesting and valuable enterprise, although it has not been without challenges and dilemmas. We have debated what chapters to include and what could have been included, as it was important to us to give breadth and meaning to the client groups and services we have chosen to portray. We wanted to ensure that the book demonstrates the value and contribution of occupational therapy, and that occupational therapy has a rightful and significant place in the services for people with mental health difficulties.

Our aim for this book was not to be wholly inclusive of all aspects of occupational therapy practice in mental health. We believe this would be an unrealistic feat given the diverse nature of mental health and social care settings and the range of opportunities which exist for occupational therapists. We wanted to use this book as a vehicle to enable some occupational therapists to share their practice and discuss how they have implemented relevant evidence where and whenever it was possible. To provide services based on sound evidence is a requirement in modern health and social care; yet it is proving to be a very real challenge – not only to practitioners but also to those who are involved with educating students. Traditional approaches to evidence-based practice do not always 'sit' comfortably with occupational therapy in mental health – so we have used definitions of evidence-based practice which go beyond research findings and include a fuller range of evidence to support clinical reasoning and decision-making.

We have tried to use real people as a means of discussing the decisions we made and how we came by them – on the understanding that these are actions which worked with that person at that time. The process as a whole was made to fit the individual, in their circumstances, given their age, life experiences, wants, needs and strengths.

Where it has not been possible to use explicit evidence this has been discussed and alternative options suggested. Occupational therapy and alternative models and theories have been proposed, together with how these can be implemented with clients in a way which is inclusive, responds to their needs and enables occupational therapists to practise in a client-centred way.

We hope that it is a valuable book to those occupational therapists, both neophyte and experienced; and that students find it a useful resource for their studies. The mental health agenda continues to change and develop. We must learn how to embrace these changes and adapt our reasoning and practice, while keeping an eye on and responding to the forces and drivers of practice.

Cathy Long
Jane Cronin-Davis

Acknowledgements

We wish to thank all our friends and colleagues who have supported us through this sometimes seemingly endless process, you know who you are, and to clients and students, who have been an unending source of inspiration and knowledge for our work in this field.

Contributors

Mandy Boaz, MSc Professional Practice, PgCert Academic Practice, DipCOT, Member of LEA, Member of the Yorkshire special interest group for learning disabilities.

Mandy originally qualified from York School of Occupational Therapy in 1979 and spent her first five years of practice working in general hospital services for older people. From 1988, she worked with people with learning disabilities, both adults and children. This work included hospital-based work but mainly involved working in community teams both as a practitioner in learning disabilities and a manager of occupational therapy services. For the last five years, Mandy has worked at York St John University College as a senior lecturer and for the last four years as Head of Programme for the BHSc (Hons) Occupational Therapy Part-time. She had a personal and voluntary interest in learning disabilities for many years and has a daughter who has a learning disability.

Sue Bower, DipOT, BSc, MSc

Sue qualified as an occupational therapist in 1979, completed a BSc (Hons) Psychology in 1990, and was awarded an MSc in Health Professional Studies in 2002. Most of Sue's occupational therapy experience has been with inter-professional, multi-agency community-based mental health teams and in related training and education roles. In recent years Sue has increasingly worked with older people living with a dementia. Since 1990 she has worked both as a practitioner and as a lecturer in health and social care. This has involved working with students of nursing, social work, physiotherapy and occupational therapy. Since November 2004, Sue has been working as a senior lecturer in the Hull School of Health and Social Care, University of Lincoln. In addition, Sue is an Advanced Dementia Care Mapper and an Approved Dementia Care Mapper Trainer with the Bradford Dementia Group, University of Bradford.

Jane Cronin-Davis, BA(Hons), BHSc(Hons), MSc (Crim Psych), PGCAP, ILT

Jane qualified in 1991 and after a short rotational post, moved in to occupational therapy in mental health, specialising in forensic mental health. She has worked in both medium and high security hospitals both as a clinician and manager. Jane currently teaches occupational therapy at Leeds Metropolitan University and has a strong interest in occupational science. She is currently researching occupational therapy practice for patients with a personality disorder diagnosis in forensic settings for her doctorate thesis.

Sarah Lloyd, SROT, MA, DipPG (Non Directive Play Therapy).

Sarah has worked in Child and Adolescent Mental Health since 1992. She has worked in a variety of settings including an in-patient unit, out-patients and intensive day treatment provision. She has also worked within education as part of an interagency pilot project looking at early identification and treatment of children at risk of becoming disaffected with education and of developing mental health issues. Her current post is as Head Occupational Therapist in the CAMHS in Fife. Postgraduate studies include an MA in Psychoanalytic Studies and a qualification in play therapy. Sarah also works as a lecturer and supervisor for the University of York on the Play Therapy training programme.

Cathy Long, SROT, DipCOT, MSc (Applied Psychology), CertHE

Cathy currently teaches at University College of York St John. She qualified as an occupational therapist in 1982, and has worked in Birmingham and Manchester as a mental health occupational therapist. She has worked in adult mental health community teams, resource centres, acute inpatient services, and a specialist unit for group psychotherapy. More recently she worked in an NHS funded arts and activities centre for people with mental health problems. She has a strong interest in women's mental health and has taken modules at master's level in related subjects.

Gill Richmond, DipCot, Grad Dip Counselling, PGDip Cognitive Therapy, BABCP accredited CBT practitioner

Gill trained at the University College of York St John and qualified as an occupational therapist in 1991. She has worked in a range of mental health settings including a community mental health team. Gill pursued further training in counselling and gained a Graduate Diploma in Counselling from the University College of York St John in 1997. She enjoyed her role as a Lecturer/Practitioner in Occupational Therapy at the York St John University College, working mainly with students on the undergraduate programme (1998–2004). She developed an interest in cognitive-behavioural therapy (CBT) and trained at the University of York and later at Newcastle Cognitive and Behavioural Therapies Centre gaining a Post-graduate Diploma in Cognitive Therapy validated by the University of Durham. She achieved accreditation as a CBT therapist in 2005. Gill currently lectures in CBT at the Department of Health Sciences at the University of York. She provides supervision to students training in CBT and continues to do clinical work one day a week. Her current title is Lecturer in Cognitive Behavioural Therapy.

Lindsay Rigby, SROT, Dip COT, BSc (Hons), MSc

Lindsay is employed as a teaching fellow at Manchester University and Manchester Mental Health & Social Care Trust as a practice development practitioner.

With over 20 years experience in occupational therapy in acute mental health, she has spent the past eight years in a Home Treatment Team offering alternatives to hospital admission. She currently specialises in the development of clinical pathways to provide cognitive-behavioural therapy and family interventions alongside specific occupational therapy interventions. Her area of specialist interest is with those who experience a first episode of psychosis and the supervision of clinicians.

Ian Wilson, RMN, Dip PSI (Thorn) BSc (Hons) MSc (COPE)

Ian works as a Dual Diagnosis Trainer and Clinical Specialist in Dual Diagnosis for Manchester Mental Health & Social Care Trust. He has worked in central Manchester for 15 years. During that time he has offered evidence-based psychosocial interventions to many clients, including CBT for individuals and their families. He has trained staff from a wide variety of backgrounds and professions in the delivery of psychosocial interventions, locally, nationally and abroad. He has a particular interest in working with young people experiencing a recent onset of psychosis and their families, and patients with complex 'dual diagnosis' presentations. He is currently also a Teaching Fellow at the University of Manchester.

Caroline Wolverson, Dip COT, Dip Horticultural Therapy, MSc Professional Practice, Certificate in Education

Caroline has worked in a variety of settings: developing an occupational therapy service to private and local authority residential and nursing homes; a two-year project facilitating effective discharge for older people with mental health problems on an acute admissions unit; and working within a community mental health team for older people. She has a particular interest in working with people with dementia and their carers living in care homes. Prior to lecturing at University College of York St John, Caroline worked in a range of clinical fields including learning disabilities and community equipment and adaptations. Since 1996 her clinical work has predominantly involved working with older people with mental health problems in both the in-patient and community settings. Her areas of particular interest are: working with people with dementia and their carers, effective communication and anxiety management.

1: Tracking developments in mental health practice

Jane Cronin-Davis and Cathy Long

This is a book for occupational therapists written primarily by occupational therapists, all with varied experience of mental health practice. It is written partly in response to requests from newly qualified occupational therapists seeking to further their skills and practice beyond the undergraduate expectations; in addition, it is a text for occupational therapy students who wish to consider how to use evidence-based practice in a field which is beginning to aspire to this. It has also been written to show readers that occupational therapy in mental health can have a significant impact on the occupational needs and strengths of the clients we come into contact with. Every chapter's authors hope to give you the benefit of their professional experience and knowledge as they explain how they would consider working with each of the clients introduced in the chapters.

A brief return to occupational therapy's roots

It is not the intention of this introductory chapter to give a complete and detailed history of the development of occupational therapy – full explanations can be found in one of the following texts: Creek (2002), Wilcock (2002), Couldrick and Aldred (2003), Duncan (2005). But it is interesting and pertinent to note that the foundations of the profession lie in the field of mental health. The introduction of occupational therapy to England during the 1920s is accredited to Dr Elizabeth Casson, who founded Dorset House in Bristol, a residential unit for female psychiatric patients, attached to which was the first occupational therapy school in England (Paterson 2002). The founding members of the profession of occupational therapy recognised that useful activity and forms of occupation helped patients with mental health difficulties, at a time when psychiatry had become more humane. The benefit for patients of structured and purposeful activity was recognised even then; but the concept of evidence-based practice was yet to come. It seemed to be sufficient to acknowledge that occupational therapy brought about change for people with mental health problems; provided structure, routine and meaning to their routines; and enabled them to maintain or develop skills and roles necessary for living.

Current influences on mental health practice

There have been major changes in service policy and provision since then. Goodwin (1997) discusses in depth the considerable policy shifts in North America and western Europe regarding mental health service provision. Initially, there was a widely accepted notion that a diverse range of community-based services was a better alternative than in-patient care in large mental health hospitals. This, Goodwin suggests, provides a more diverse spectrum of care and is being recognised as necessary provision. Mental health services now commonly provide: mental health units within general hospitals, day hospitals, secure provision, primary care services and community teams.

Recently in the UK, a surge of government guidelines and documents have profoundly influenced the way mental health services have been developed and delivered nationally. Consequently, there has been a shift in the ways occupational therapists work at both a client–therapist level and at a broader service level: we now work in ways very different from those of our predecessors, which brings both challenges and opportunities. *Cases for Change*, published in 2004 (National Institute for Mental Health in England (NIMHE 2004a)), states that mental health services in England are going through a period of 'unprecedented change' and highlights important policy changes. It states that the mental health policy of the twenty-first century includes a diverse range of issues namely, building effective services; vulnerability and risk; managing mental health symptoms and promoting well-being. Equally important are the issues relating to user involvement and social inclusion. It is beyond the remit of this book to consider and discuss these policy changes in depth, however, it would be remiss not to highlight these key initiatives with regard to our current and future practice.

In 1991, the Care Programme Approach (CPA) was introduced. CPA guarantees that people who come under the remit of specialist mental health services are assessed, have a care plan and care co-ordinator, and have regular reviews. Supervision registers came into force in 1994 (NIMHE 2004a) for those people who were considered to be especially vulnerable. Following this the Mental Health (Patients in the Community) Act 1995 allowed the supervised discharge of patients in the community. The white paper, *Modernising Mental Health Services: Safe, Sound and Supportive* (Department of Health (DoH) 1998a) emphasised the need for robust comprehensive care (looking at gaps in services); bed provision (secure and 24 hour care); and assertive outreach and crisis teams. Further key strategies have been produced by the government to ensure more accountability in the way services are provided for those with mental health problems: *A First Class Service* (DoH 1998b) instituted the systems of clinical governance, standard setting, professional accountability and monitoring, focusing National Health Service (NHS) professionals on providing high-quality services. In 1999, a landmark initiative was introduced entitled the *National Service Framework for Mental Health* (DoH 1999). This NSF comprises seven standards which focus on different aspects of care and includes performance indicators. Additional NSFs aimed at addressing the needs of children (DoH 2004) and older people (DoH 2001a) are relevant to the focus of this book. With regard to children, the NSF states that there needs to be an improvement in services, multi-disciplinary working and access to evidence-based care for the mental health and psychological well-being of children and young people. The NSF for older people states that services must promote mental health, and support older people with depression and dementia.

Further planning for mental health provision over a ten-year period is included in *The NHS Plan* (DoH 2000). The changes in service delivery include 1000 graduate mental health workers; a further 500 community mental health team staff; 50 early intervention teams for young people with psychosis; 335 crisis resolution teams; a total of 220 assertive outreach teams; women-only services; an extra 700 staff to work with carers; services for prisoners with mental health problems, including care plans and key workers for every prisoner with mental illness who leaves prison; and suitable service provision for approximately 400 patients in the high secure hospitals (NIMHE 2004a). The proposals outlined in *The NHS Plan* and the NSF for mental health, have been further emphasised in the *Mental Health Policy Implementation Guide* (DoH 2001b). The guide offers comprehensive descriptions of service models for different components of mental health provision. One of its key messages is that these new initiatives require new ways of working, with staff who are equipped with the 'right range of competencies'.

Scotland has its own Mental Health (Care and Treatment) (Scotland) Act 2003. The Scottish Executive Policy for Mental Health is working towards the mental well-being of the people in Scotland, and improving the situations of those with mental ill-health. Work is in progress to promote attitudes and behaviour in the general public which lead to mental well-being; and to ensure that good quality mental health services are available for everyone who needs them, at all levels of need. The policy will address laws relating to mental health; restricted patients; NHS aspects of mental health and well-being (see www.scotland.gov. uk/Topics/Health/care/15216/15052).

A further recent development includes clinical guidelines produced by the National Institute for Health and Clinical Excellence including recommended intervention for anxiety (NICE 2004a), depression (NICE 2004b), eating disorders (NICE 2004c), schizophrenia (NICE 2002), depression in young people (NICE 2005a) and obsessive-compulsive disorder (NICE 2005b). These are specific clinical guidelines which appraise the research and evidence base, and provide direct recommendations as to the most appropriate care and treatment relevant to the clinical condition.

Some may find that the modernisation of mental health services is both considerable and daunting. However, the key messages are: to provide a wide range of effective, comprehensive services which are based on sound principles and what is considered to work. These policies and documents all influence how mental health services should be delivered and provide evidence to support occupational therapy practice.

Evidence-based practice: a necessary component?

Measuring outcomes and evidence-based practice are terms which have become common parlance in today's health and social care arena, and are clearly expectations of current professional practice. Herbert *et al.* (2001) suggest that actively searching, selecting, appraising and applying research evidence in practice is a requirement for all the health professions. Sackett and colleagues (1996) are accredited with the definition of evidence-based medicine:

> 'The conscientious, explicit and judicious use of the current best evidence about the care of individual patients.'

There has been, however, an assumption that evidence based on research findings is the only worthwhile evidence, especially that from a quantitative tradition (Rycroft-Malone *et al.* 2004). A given and widely accepted hierarchy of evidence (Table 1.1) is the one provided by the NSF for mental health (DoH 1999).

Rycroft-Malone *et al.* (2004) state that there has been considerable expenditure and philosophical effort regarding the 'evidence-based practice agenda'. They argue that although we should as practitioners deliver care based on what works, challenges remain about what the evidence is and how it can be used given the actualities of clinical practice. Is it perhaps more beneficial to consider the notion of evidence-based practice as postulated by Higgs and Jones (2000), which is knowledge that has been derived from a variety of sources, been tested, and has found to be credible. Is this more preferable and acceptable to the busy practitioner? Rycroft-Malone *et al.* argue that to practice person-centred care which is indeed evidence based, practitioners need to consider and integrate: research; clinical experience; patient, client and carer experiences; and the local context and environment (Figure 1.1). The call now, they suggest, is to use the necessary approaches and multiple sources of knowledge relevant to a particular clinical problem.

This could provide a useful framework for evidence-based occupational therapy today; negligible research exists for different areas of occupational therapy: mental health is a real example (Duncan 2005). Given our clear emphasis on client-centred

Table 1.1 Bandolier hierarchy of evidence as cited in the NSF for mental health (1999).

Level	Type of research evidence
Type I evidence	At least one good systematic review, including at least one randomised controlled trial
Type II evidence	At least one good randomised controlled trial
Type III evidence	At least one well-designed intervention study without randomisation
Type IV evidence	At least one well-designed observational study
Type V evidence	Expert opinion, including the opinion of service users and carers

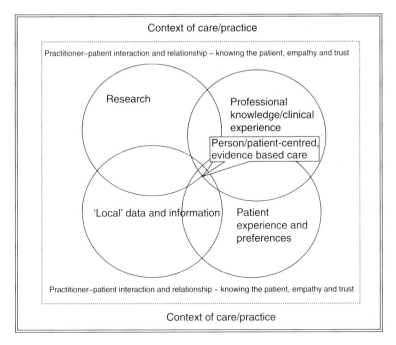

Figure 1.1 Four sources of evidence for patient-centred, evidence-based practice. Reproduced from Rycroft-Malone *et al.* (2004) What counts as evidence in evidence-based practice? *Journal of Advanced Nursing.* **47**: 81–90, with permission from Blackwell Publishing.

practice, perhaps doggedly pursuing quantitative research findings and methods is inappropriate – a more collective or holistic method as outlined above might be more useful to both client and practitioner. In a similar vein, Hyde (2004) emphasises the client-centred nature of occupational therapy and endorses research methods which can harness the complex inter-relationships between therapist, client and intervention. Yet as has been suggested, randomised controlled trials remain the gold standard by which effectiveness of treatments is measured.

What about values?

More promisingly, there is increasing acknowledgement of the place of values in health care as a balance to evidence-based practice. In fact the US Institute of Medicine (2001) definition of evidence-based practice refers to the integration of best research evidence with clinical expertise and patient values (cited in Azrin and Goldman 2005). Clinical expertise in occupational therapy could refer to using our own clinical and past expertise to identify and make judgements about a person's occupational needs; interests and strengths; his/her readiness/current capacity to engage with occupational therapy. The third strand to evidence-based practice – patient values – underlines the importance of patients' preferences for health care. What do they value? This necessitates making informed choices, and those choices being respected. This calls for everyone involved in health and social care, including occupational therapists, to be able to articulate their purpose and potential value, ideally with reference to evidence.

In the UK there is a growing interest in 'values-based practice' in mental heath as the means by which values can be scrutinised more closely to enhance quality of service to our users (Woodridge and Fulford 2004). Thus recognising that the values and attitudes which both clients and mental health workers bring influence the quality of health and social care received. This necessarily turns the spotlight onto subjective experience, while appraising the evidence is a more objective process. For further information on value-orientated services see the NIMHE Values Framework (2004b).

NIMHE (2004b) recognises values alongside evidence in all areas of mental health policy and practice and in its framework of values for mental health is concerned with raising awareness of values involved in different contexts; and of respecting different values. Its primary concern is with the centrality of each individual service user and their communities to the decisions undertaken by professionals.

How to use this book

As you may have already surmised the contributors to this book have taken a wider definition of evidence-based practice than the one referred to in Table 1.1. We have used people from our own practice as a basis for illustrating the ways in which theory, research evidence, government guidelines and client centred practice can be used to inform our clinical reasoning and intervention. Each chapter focuses on a different area of mental health and tries to show how the occupational therapy process might apply with an individual in that particular context.

Inevitably, contributors bring differences in practice based on each client's diagnosis, needs, values, and social and temporal contexts. Clinical reasoning is also influenced by differences in professional experience, post-graduate training, the mental health setting and the available evidence base. No contributor provides one definitive answer for each person – as such we hope to avoid falling into the trap of writing recipes for specific conditions. This is not a manual for occupational therapy practice in mental health, as with all current recommendations for health and social care, the outlined interventions are individually tailored. One size does not fit all! This practice has long been recognised as good occupational therapy and is a core part of our philosophy.

To maintain client confidentiality pseudonyms have been used throughout and in some cases details have been changed to prevent any possibility of identification.

Each chapter includes tasks for the reader: reflective questions or suggested reading to prompt you to look beyond the confines of the book and to develop your reasoning skills. The people we discuss are presented in a sequence across the life span, starting with children through to older adults, but adults of working age dominate. However, this is perhaps offset by the range of people, their life experiences, occupations, diagnoses, and the theoretical approaches and intervention settings.

Briefly, the content of each chapter is as follows:

Chapter 2: It's like having Tigger in the classroom

Sarah Lloyd
Attention deficit hyperactivity disorder (ADHD) is a condition that affects a significant group of children, and which has psycho-social consequences for both children and parents. This chapter focuses on the impact on one child and his family, and the role of the occupational therapist as part of a child and adolescent mental health team. Case studies are used to illustrate the efficacy of a range of therapies, with special focus on helping the child to manage his feelings.

Chapter 3: Enhancing self-efficacy in managing major depression

Gill Richmond
Occupational therapy in mental health integrates evidence-based strategies to facilitate a clear understanding of the individual environmental, socio-cultural, cognitive, emotional and behavioural factors leading to the development and maintenance of depression. This case study provides opportunity for reflection on strategies which guide the therapist's clinical reasoning and will assist collaborative implementation of the most suitable and effective therapeutic interventions for the person experiencing depression. Reference is made to guidelines on the treatment of depression formulated by NICE (2004b).

Chapter 4: Occupational therapy interventions for someone experiencing severe and enduring mental illness

Lindsay Rigby and Ian Wilson
Adhering closely to principles of evidence-based practice, this chapter gives a detailed account of 'psycho-social interventions' (PSI) for schizophrenia. Training in PSI is usually at the post-graduate level and multi-disciplinary, and it is becoming increasingly recognised as treatment of choice – hence its inclusion here. Using the Canadian Occupational Performance Measure (Law *et al.* 1990) as a starting point, Linzi and Ian show how the symptoms of schizophrenia affect 'Bob's' ability to engage with his previous occupations and with his family. They then describe detailed and clearly defined interventions to help Bob and his family to meet their goals.

Chapter 5: Not drowning but waving: working with female survivors of childhood sexual abuse

Cathy Long

This is not a traditional area of focus for occupational therapy, reflected by the limited reference to the needs of survivors of childhood sexual abuse (CSA) in the occupational therapy literature. However the possible impact of childhood sexual abuse on health and psycho-social function is well documented elsewhere, including the high incidence of survivors in adult mental health services. The first part of the chapter gives an introduction to these issues, in addition to general principles relevant to working with women who have been abused. This is followed by discussion of occupational therapy. The Kawa (river) model (Iwama 2005) is used as the means to begin working with 'Karen'.

Chapter 6: Personality disorder: occupational therapy inclusion

Jane Cronin-Davis

This chapter addresses how the occupational therapy process can be applied in a forensic setting, while taking into account the legal implications and potential restrictions on occupational therapy practice. It discusses the role of the occupational therapist when working with someone who is considered challenging in terms of their presentation and behaviour.

Issues such as occupational alienation, deprivation and disruption are all considered in relation to Joe. Jane acknowledges the paucity of research evidence to support occupational therapy interventions, yet demonstrates how occupational therapy intervention must be a core component of the multi-disciplinary assessment and treatment process on a specialist in-patient unit for people diagnosed as having personality disorder.

Chapter 7: Dual diagnosis: learning disabilities and dementia. Working towards ensuring people with a dual diagnosis receive quality services

Mandy Boaz

As stated in *Valuing People: A Strategy for Learning Disability for the 21st Century* (DoH 2001c) people with learning disabilities are more likely to experience mental illness and are more prone to chronic health problems than the general population. 'David' lives in his own home and has Down's syndrome, and, as is often the case, he has developed dementia, which has added to the complexity of his needs. Discussion of occupational therapy with David is underpinned by government initiatives and is used as a means of informing and supporting clinical reasoning. Reed and Sanderson's (1999) 'Adaptation through occupation model' is used to guide thinking and practice.

Chapter 8: Working with John Lane: a person-centred approach to supporting the person with dementia and their carers

Caroline Wolverson

John Lane has a diagnosis of vascular dementia and lives in a residential home. Caroline discusses the steps involved in working as an occupational therapist with John, while remaining closely faithful to the principles of person-centred practice and multi-disciplinary working. Consideration of his physical needs (John also has arthritis) and pressures arising from residential living is included, together with possible strategies for managing both of these areas. References to evidence to support suggested interventions are made with a particular focus on life story work and environmental adaptation.

We recommend that Chapters 8 and 9 are read in conjunction with each other.

Chapter 9: Exploring lived experiences of occupational therapy and dementia

Sue Bower

This chapter also uses person-centred practice as the primary focus for discussion of a person's experience of dementia. Unlike John, Alice lives alone, and is causing concern for her daughter. Sue takes us through a process of questioning traditional knowledge, and understanding and practice in this area so that we are better able to appreciate differing perceptions of Alice's situation – ours, the reader is only one of many! Key themes are engagement and inclusion, well-being, occupational performance and risk with discussion of implications for occupational therapy in each of these areas. Sue acknowledges the complexity of what it is like to live with dementia, and that effective person-centred practice necessarily involves multi-faceted reasoning and decision-making.

Summary

This book is intended for occupational therapy students studying in the UK and abroad. It will also benefit qualified occupational therapists, principally those on rotation or those who have not yet decided on a clinical speciality, who wish to examine and qualify existing practice. In addition it will benefit other health care students and qualified health professionals who will be challenged to base all practice on sound evidence rather than anecdotal experience.

The book may not provide all of the answers, but will, hopefully, as a starting point steer readers in a direction where they can think about and reason how to best provide effective interventions to those who are in need of mental health services. It could also help occupational therapists to redefine their practice and consider occupation-focused occupational therapy. We recognise that the call for evidence-based practice is strong and unrelenting, and we can as a profession address this given the clear direction resources and experiences.

References

Azrin, S.T. and Goldman, H.H. (2005) Evidence based practice emerges. In: Drake, R.E., Merrens, M.R. and Lynde, D.W. (eds) *Evidence-Based Mental Health Practice*. London: WW Norton & Company.

Couldrick, L. and Aldred, D. (2003) *Forensic Occupational Therapy*. London: Whurr Publishers.

Creek, J. (2002) *Occupational Therapy and Mental Health*, 3rd edn. London: Churchill Livingstone.

DoH (1998a) *Modernising Mental Health Services: Safe, Sound and Supportive*. London: Department of Health.

DoH (1998b) *A First Class Service*. London: Department of Health.

DoH (2000) *The NHS Plan*. London: Department of Health.

DoH (1999) *National Service Framework for Mental Health*. London: Department of Health.

DoH (2001a) *National Service Framework for Older People*. London: Department of Health.

DoH (2001b) *Mental Health Policy Implementation Guide*. London: Department of Health.

DoH (2001c) *Valuing People: A Strategy for Learning Disability for the 21st Century*. London: Department of Health.

DoH (2004) *National Service Framework for Children, Young People and Maternity Services*. London: Department of Health.

Duncan, E. (ed.) (2005) *Foundations for Practice in Occupational Therapy*, 4th edn. Edinburgh: Elsevier Churchill Livingstone.

Goodwin, S. (1997) *Comparative Mental Health Policy: From Institutional to Community Care*. London: Sage.

Herbert, R.D., Sherrington, C., Maher, C. and Moseley, A.M. (2001) Evidence-based practice – imperfect but necessary. *Physiotherapy Theory and Practice*. **17**: 201–11.

Higgs, J. and Jones, M. (2000) *Clinical Reasoning in the Health Professions*, 2nd edn. Oxford: Botterworth Heinemann.

Hyde, P. (2004) Fool's gold: examining the use of gold standards in the production of research evidence. *British Journal of Occupational Therapy*. **67**: 89–94.

Institute of Medicine (2001) Crossing the quality chasm: A new health system for the 21st century. Washington DC: National Academy Press, quoted in: Azrin, S.T. and Goldman, H.H. (2005) Evidence-based practice emerges. In: Drake, R.E., Merrens, M.R. and Lynde, D.W. (eds) *Evidence-Based Mental Health Practice*. New York: W.W. Norton.

Iwama, M. (2005) The Kawa Model; nature, life flow, and the power of culturally relevant occupational therapy. Duncan, E. (ed.) *Foundations for Practice in Occupational Therapy*, 4th edn. Edinburgh: Elsevier Churchill Livingstone, pp. 213–31.

Law, M., Baptiste, S., McColl, M., Opzoomer, A., Polatajko, H. and Pollock, N. (1990) Canadian Occupational Performance Measure: An outcome measure for Occupational Therapy. *Canadian Journal of Occupational Therapy*. **57**: 82–7.

Mental Health (Care and Treatment) (Scotland) Act 2003. Available at: www.opsi.gov.uk/legislation/scotland/acts2003/20030013.htm [accessed 11/02/2006].

NICE (2002) *Schizophrenia: Core Interventions in the Treatment and Management of Schizophrenia in Primary and Secondary Care*. London: National Institute for Clinical Excellence. Available at: www.nice.org.uk/page.aspx?o=42424 [accessed 12/02/2006].

NICE (2004a) *Anxiety: Management of Anxiety (Panic Disorder, With or Without Agoraphobia, and Generalised Anxiety Disorder) in Adults in Primary, Secondary and Community Care*. London: National Institute for Clinical Excellence. Available at: www.nice.org.uk/page.aspx?o=235216 [accessed 12/02/2006].

NICE (2004b) *Depression: Management of Depression in Primary and Secondary Care*. London: National Institute for Clinical Excellence. Available at: www.nice.org.uk/page.aspx?o=235213 [accessed 12/02/2006].

NICE (2004c) *Eating Disorders: Core Interventions in the Treatment and Management of Anorexia Nervosa, Bulimia Nervosa and Related Eating Disorders*. London: National Institute for Clinical Excellence. Available at: www.nice.org.uk/page.aspx?o=101239 [accessed 12/02/2006].

NICE (2005a) *Depression in Children and Young People: Identification and Management in Primary, Community and Secondary Care*. London: National Institute for Health and Clinical Excellence. Available at: www.nice.org.uk/page.aspx?o=273073 [accessed 12/02/2006].

NICE (2005b) *Obsessive Compulsive Disorder: Core interventions in the treatment of obsessive compulsive disorder and body dysmorphic disorder*. London: National Institute for Health and Clinical Excellence. Available at: www.nice.org.uk/page.aspx?o=276850 [accessed 12/02/2006].

NIMHE (2004a) *Cases for Change*. London: National Institute for Mental Health in England.

NIMHE (2004b) *Values for Mental Health*. Available at: http://kc.nimhe.org.uk/upload/NIMHE%20Values%20Framework.pdf [accessed 06/02/2006].

Paterson, C. (2002) A short history of occupational therapy. In: Creek, J. (ed.) *Occupational Therapy and Mental Health* (3rd edn). Edinburgh: Churchill Livingstone.

Reed, K. and Sanderson, S. (1999) *Concepts of Occupational Therapy*, 4th edn. Philadelphia: Lippincott Williams and Wilkins.

Rycroft-Malone, J., Seers, K., Titchen, A., Harvey, G., Kitson, A. and McCormack, B. (2004) What counts as evidence in evidence-based practice? *Journal of Advanced Nursing*. **47**: 81–90.

Sackett, D.L., Rosenberg, W.M.C., Gray, J.A.M., Haynes, R.B. and Richardson, W.S. (1996) Evidence-based medicine: what it is and what it isn't. *British Medical Journal*. **312**: 71–2.

Wilcock, A. (2002) *Occupation for Health, Volume 2*. London: British Association of Occupational Therapy.

Woodridge, K. and Fulford, K.W.M. (2004) *Whose Values. A work book for values-based practice in mental health care*. London: The Sainsbury Centre for Mental Health.

2: It's like having Tigger in the classroom

Sarah Lloyd

Theory into practice 1

Gavin was 5 years old and coming to the end of his first year at primary school when his teacher asked for help. She had many years' experience in early years education but was baffled by Gavin and felt 'de-skilled' that her wealth of strategies and experience in helping children with difficulties had failed to have any significant impact on Gavin's behaviour. Initially she had thought that he was probably just a bit immature and would grow out of his difficulties, but things just seemed to be getting worse.

Gavin struggled to sit on the carpet at story time without fidgeting and squirming in a way that was disruptive to the whole class. This also meant that someone else often came into contact with Gavin's hands or feet. When the children were supposed to be working in small groups Gavin was invariably wandering round the classroom. Even when the teaching assistant was sitting right next to him, the teacher could see that he wasn't really listening and was looking around, jigging up and down in his chair, playing with the things on the table. Things in the playground were no better, and Gavin always got into trouble for pushing or hitting other children or just being where he wasn't supposed to be. His friendships never seemed to last and the other children were becoming fed up with him. In spite of all this she could not help liking him; he was a delightful little boy who was always sorry when he was told off and seemed to want to be good but somehow never quite managed it.

The teacher also felt that she had lost her relationship with mum who no longer came in person to collect her son. Mum said that she couldn't face the 'playground mafia' of other mums and dreaded their comments ('Your son hit my boy today for no reason'; 'You need to get a grip on that boy') and the inevitable summons by the teacher to hear about Gavin's misdemeanours of that day.

Attention deficit hyperactivity disorder (ADHD), or hyperkinetic syndrome as it is often known in the UK, is a condition that affects between 3% and 5% of the population (DSM-IV – APA 1994). Three to six times as many boys as girls are diagnosed with ADHD (Whalen 1989). It is always present before the age of 7 years, usually before the age of 5 and often before the age of 2. It often lasts into adulthood and is characterised by inattention, hyperactivity and impulsivity to such a degree that the child's psychological development is significantly impaired (Taylor *et al.* 2004). It is a complex disorder steeped in co-morbidities that are most effectively assessed and treated by a multi-disciplinary team (NICE 2000). There is no empirical evidence to show the benefit of occupational therapy for children with ADHD, but this does not mean that occupational therapists are not making a significant contribution or that their practice is not founded on sound theory and clinical judgement.

Chu (2003) conducted a national survey of mainly paediatric occupational therapists to gauge the level of involvement with children with ADHD. Of the 30% of therapists who replied 63% had children with ADHD on their caseload. Paediatric occupational therapists working with children with ADHD tended to use a sensory integrative approach (Mangeot *et al.* 2001, Chu 2003). Within the scope of this book, this chapter will outline interventions most commonly used by occupational therapists in child and adolescent mental health teams. Sensory integration techniques tend to be used more by occupational therapists in paediatrics although, as I will discuss later, it would be useful to study a combined approach.

ADHD – assessment and diagnosis

The International Classification of Diseases 10th edition (ICD 10) criteria for ADHD are that all three conditions of inattention, impulsivity and hyperactivity should be present to a clinically significant level, occurring at a severity and frequency that significantly effect the child's ability to function at home, at school and in their peer group. If the condition is untreated it can lead to delinquency and other antisocial behaviour, underachievement at school (Taylor *et al.* 2004), and in the work place (Klein and Menuzza, 1991) and difficulties in making and sustaining meaningful relationships (Wenar 1994).

In understanding the role of occupational therapy with these children we must look at the context in which assessment and treatment is delivered – that of the multi-disciplinary team.

Assessment

The multi-disciplinary team usually comprises professionals from psychiatry and/or paediatrics, psychology and nursing, and sometimes social work, occupational therapy, child psychotherapy, speech and language therapy. The task of the team assessing the child and family presenting with ADHD is a complex one. There are other conditions that share some features of ADHD (e.g. an anxious or depressed child may appear distracted and agitated, a child with undiagnosed hearing difficulties may have trouble hearing what the teacher is saying and seem distracted and inattentive) but it is the frequency and severity of the combination of symptoms that are crucial in the diagnosis of ADHD. The assessment should consist of the parts covered below, and ideally the child should be seen in at least two settings (e.g. clinic and school).

Interview with parents

This is usually carried out by a child psychiatrist or paediatrician and includes a detailed medical history (from conception through early developmental milestones – psychological and physiological) as well as specific questions concerning the symptoms of ADHD and those of related difficulties (Taylor *et al.* 2004). It is important to exclude other possible causes for the child's difficulties and understand the family context in which the difficulties are occurring – both genetic and environmental.

Interview with the child

Children over the age of about 5 years can give a good picture of how they see themselves and how they feel they are managing at home, at school and in their relationships with their peers. Occupational therapists carrying out this part of the assessment should remember that children often play things out in the way that grown-ups talk things through (Wilson *et al.* 1992, Jennings 1995, West 1996). They can use play, drama or art activities to help the child express and explore these themes. Giving the child concrete tools with which they can illustrate themselves and their environment may elicit a lot more information than, for instance, asking a child to talk about their family.

The therapist tries to make an assessment of the child including concentration, application to task, social disinhibition, level of activity, self-esteem and any emotional difficulties. It is important to observe the way in which a child carries out an instruction. Are they anxious and fretful? Are they over confident and start before the therapist has finished giving instructions? Do they start the task but then have a different idea and move on to doing their own thing? Do they keep checking if they are doing it right – either verbally or by looking at the therapist to try to gauge the latter's reaction?

Theory into practice 2

I brought a large box of assorted animals to the first assessment session with Gavin. I asked him to choose one animal to represent himself in the family and to put it in the middle of the paper. Gavin chose a fierce looking lion then changed it to an equally wild looking tiger. I then asked Gavin to choose animals to be the other people in his family. Gavin carefully chose a range of farm animals – cows and horses – to be his mother, father, brother and sister. Gavin placed these animals together at the other side of the page to himself. As he did this Gavin explained that he wasn't really like them, they were more 'normal' and things didn't keep going wrong with them, things just went 'right'. I then asked Gavin to arrange the animals to show who got on best with whom in the family. Gavin put his mum and dad close together and he and his mum close to each other. His brother and sister were slightly further away. He was then asked if he could make one change to the family what would he change. Gavin delved back into the box of animals and found a horse and swapped his tiger for a horse, so he could be more normal and like the rest of them. He also moved all the animals so that they were closer to each other and started playing out a game with them all.

Self-assessments can be useful in older children. From about the age of 9 children often enjoy completing questionnaires asking them about the different areas of their lives and how they feel about things (e.g. Conners' self-assessment (Conners 1989) or the child self-report, (Achenbach 1991). Below this age children struggle with the reading and comprehension requirements of these forms and most information has to be gleaned from observing the child in different situations – at home, at school, at play.

The interpretation of the individual assessment can be difficult because many children with ADHD can mange this 1:1 situation reasonably well (especially if the room is relatively free from distractions and the child has the undivided attention of one adult); as such it is important that this forms only part of the assessment.

School visit and liaison

School visits are only done with the express permission of the parents. Direct observation of the child in school is the best possible assessment. Such observation allows the clinician to make an assessment of the child's level of functioning in a challenging environment as well as assessment of the teacher – child interaction, the environment of the classroom and ethos of the school. It is useful to observe the child in the structured environment of the classroom and the relatively unstructured times of play time and lunchtime. It is generally most effective if the child does not know that they are being observed. School observation is a role that is often carried out by occupational therapists who use their skills in observation and activity analysis to good effect. Where direct observation is not possible, standardised questionnaires (e.g. Conners scales for teachers (Conners 1989), child behaviour checklists (Achenbach 1991)) and subsequent telephone discussions with a member of the assessment team may be used. For example, in the Conners questionnaire the teacher completes a series of questions about the child and their behaviour and attitude in the classroom. When scored, this breaks the child's difficulties into the sorts of problems that are likely to indicate a conduct disorder, those which are more indicative of learning difficulties, or those more commonly associated with hyperactivity or ADHD. The teacher's questionnaire is then compared with the parent's questionnaire and, in older children, the self-assessment. The results of all these help to inform the assessment team, but these should not be used in place of direct observation and assessment.

▓ Theory into practice 3 ▓

In Gavin's 40-minute classroom observation, he was seen to be much more active in and around the classroom than his peers, He left his seat about every 30 seconds to go to another part of the classroom – borrowing a pencil, chatting to a friend, or looking at what was happening out of the window. When he was sitting in his seat he was constantly on the move on his seat – swinging on it, tapping his legs and feet, swirling around to see what was happening behind him. With the teaching assistant sitting right next to him he needed constant prompting to stay on task. Even with this he failed to carry out the problem-solving task that was being discussed. His level of distraction was such that he did not seem to process verbal instructions that were longer than one succinct sentence.

The assessor noticed that the other children in the class frequently 'told tales' to the teacher about what Gavin was doing so there was a lot of highlighting of his difficult behaviour in the course of the afternoon. He was not allowed to sit on the carpet at story time because his constant squirming and fidgeting distracted the other children and invariably led to children being hit and kicked.

At afternoon playtime he had to stand with the playground supervisor rather than play with his friends because of an incident that had happened at lunchtime. The playground supervisor said the he was the one child who appeared most frequently in her 'little book' and didn't know what to do with him.

Gavin's classmates seemed to quite like him on one level and enjoyed having fun with him but quickly became frustrated with him and his constantly getting into trouble and changing things.

The Conners teachers rating scale (Conners 1989) showed high scores in the inattention, hyperactivity and ADHD sub scales and a low score in the oppositional behaviour sub scale.

Psychometric testing

The team may use some standardised assessment tools (e.g. Conners 1989) but these should be backed up with direct observation and interviews. Psychometric testing by psychologists may be useful in measuring the child's academic potential against their actual performance at school. There are also tests of executive functioning that have been developed (Sergeant et al. 2002) which can be useful in assessment and diagnosis. Barkley (1991) suggests that a limitation of these can be that the laboratory results often fail to be accurately reproduced in 'real' settings. Again this reinforces the importance of an assessment comprising a range of tools.

Diagnosis

Gathering all this information can be a lengthy process. The psychologist may have completed a psychometric assessment, there may have been a home visit, perhaps by a member of the nursing team, the occupational therapist may have made an assessment of the child and a visit to school, the child psychiatrist or paediatrician may have done a developmental assessment, the paediatrician may have done a medical examination. Once all the strands of the assessment are complete the team can meet and use the information gathered to inform the doctor within the team and help him/her to make an accurate diagnosis. Once agreement about a diagnosis has been reached discussion about the most appropriate package of treatment for the child and family can begin.

Concomitant factors

There is a high level of co-morbidity with ADHD (e.g. conduct disorder) (Gillberg et al. 2004). This will have been considered as part of the assessment but it is important to be aware of compounding and complicating factors when working with children and families with ADHD. Concomitant factors include:

- *Conduct disorder.* Although there can be some similarities in presentation (e.g. inadequate self-control) these are different conditions (Fergusson *et al.* 1991) with distinct aetiology and require different treatment.
- *Emotional disorders.* Anxiety, depression, low self-esteem and insecurity may follow the failures at school, home and friendships.
- *Specific learning difficulties.* Children with ADHD are more likely to show specific neurodevelopmental delays (Semud-Clikeman *et al.* 1992).
- *Developmental co-ordination delay* (DCD). This is often seen in terms of poor hand writing, clumsiness, poor performance in sport and delay in reaching developmental milestones (Gillberg 2000).

The presence or absence of any or all of these will obviously influence the decision of the team about which treatment approaches will be most effective.

Treatment

Medication

One major strand of treatment is often medication (methylphenidate, dexamfetamine). These stimulants quickly and effectively reduce the impulsiveness, restlessness and inattention of the child and so improve their capacity for social interaction and improve compliance (Taylor *et al.* 2004). They are not a cure for ADHD but can work to reduce the impact of the disorder. Some stimulants (e.g. methylphenidate) have an effect that lasts only a few hours whereas others (OROS methylphenidate) are longer acting. These are important considerations for the clinician and doctor to discuss in relation to the school day and the relationship between the family and school. An advantage of the short-acting nature of the medication is that families can have breaks from the medication at weekends or in school holidays if desired. There is much, well-documented evidence for the use and limitations of medication (see Taylor *et al.* 2004, for a summary of trials, NICE 2000, SIGN 2001). Stimulant medication has been shown to be effective in between 70% and 80%, reducing impulsive behaviour and improving concentration. This not only helps children with school work, but also improves social relationships.

Some parents are reluctant to permit the use of stimulant medicines with their child, especially if the child is young. It should be noted that there can be medical side-effects, e.g. on rate of physical development and sleep pattern. Serious consideration must be also given to the environment in which the young person is living and associating before prescribing, e.g. giving amfetamines to an adolescent on the fringes of an antisocial/drug culture may lead to misuse.

Study task 1

There are a few studies on the long-term effects of stimulant medication (Gillberg *et al.* 1997, Jensen 2002). There is a general reticence in Europe for prescribing medication to younger children. This is different from the situation in the USA, where medication is used more widely and with younger children. Parents seeking advice on this issue have often extensively read the literature available on the internet. One difficulty with this is the availability of opinions with little or no evidence, but which can be very emotionally charged. As a therapist working with children with ADHD it is important to be aware of the debates. A useful task would be to compare information available on the internet with evidence from peer-reviewed journals. One starting point for this could be Bramble's (2003) opinion on different patterns of prescribing.

Work with the family

Theory into practice 4

By the time Gavin's family came to the assessment clinic, family relationships were strained. His siblings were fed up of having their games spoiled and their toys broken. His parents felt guilty about how much time they were forced to spend with him to the detriment of the other children. They felt blamed by other parents and grandparents, all of whom had their own ideas about what should be done to 'sort that child out'. Even as a 2-year-old the strategies that had succeeded with their older children failed to make any difference to Gavin's behaviour.

The parents had stopped Gavin going out to play because they couldn't bear the constant accusations of the neighbours and their opinions about things Gavin was supposed to have done.

Gavin's parents found it almost impossible to go out as a couple because they had exhausted the friends and relatives who were willing to baby-sit if Gavin was in the house. The strain of living under such unrelenting stress was taking its toll.

Families need ongoing support and help, both in terms of information about the condition and behavioural work around managing the child within the family (Horn *et al.* 1990, 1991, Pelham *et al.* 1999). The occupational therapist most often offers help and advice around managing the child's behaviour and setting up routines and structures at home. Children with ADHD respond well to predictability and a well-structured environment (Green and Chee 1994).

Theory into practice 5

With Gavin and his family working out a morning routine, breaking down tasks in to small, achievable steps meant that mornings became less fraught and Gavin arrived at school in a much more positive frame of mind, having already been successful at home that morning. These can be very simple interventions. For Gavin and his family it was breaking down the task of 'getting ready for school' because although Gavin was always awake early and had lots of energy for the day, he was constantly getting distracted and side-tracked in the next hour so that he was rarely ready in time to leave for school.

Table 2.1 The morning routine.

Task	Boundaries and benefits
Getting up	Getting out of bed first time dad called – dad stayed with Gavin in his room until he was up
Putting on the school uniform that mum had laid out the night before	No negotiation or possible confusion about what to wear. Clear division of responsibility; mum puts the uniform out, Gavin puts it on
Sitting at the table and eating breakfast	Dad put Gavin's breakfast on the table for him (again no negotiation about what was for breakfast – all been agreed the night before). Dad sat with Gavin and ate his breakfast at the same time. No television on, toys or reading during breakfast. (Removing distractions helped Gavin to stay focused on the task. Similarly, it made it easier if dad or mum ate at the same time)
Cleaning teeth, brushing hair and putting shoes on	Again these activities were graded to ensure they are pitched at the right level for the child to succeed. In the early stages mum would put the toothbrush out with the toothpaste already on it. In the next stage mum would leave them both out but the toothpaste wasn't on the brush. Finally Gavin was able to get them out himself, brush his teeth and put them away again.
Choosing a toy or watching television	When Gavin had completed all the above tasks (a star chart to mark off the successful steps along the way was useful here) he could choose something to do until it was time to go to school

This kind of structuring of a routine is a balance between changing the environment to maximise the chances of success (giving mum and dad clear tasks as well as the child) and helping the child to take responsibility for tasks. It is relatively simple but can have a profound impact on the mood and behaviour of the whole family and certainly made a significant difference to how Gavin was when he first arrived at school in the morning. This level of activity analysis is a core skill of occupational therapists and can usefully be applied to many areas of life of the child with ADHD, at home and at school.

Other family orientated interventions involve specific teaching of strategies to manage the child's behaviour and improve the quality of the parent–child relationship. There are many different programmes although not all are based on the widely available empirical evidence about their relative efficacy (e.g. Dumas 1989, Pisterman *et al.* 1989, Kadzin 1991). It is important to weigh the evidence about different aspects of the programme, e.g. the use of modelling and role play within parenting interventions – Knapp and Deluty (1989) compared programmes that used reading and discussion with those that used modelling and role play. They found that those that used modelling and role play had a greater impact on the parenting skills of the participants.

Study task 2

Behavioural family interventions form a large part of the work of child and adolescent mental health teams. They are many and varied and it would be useful for the student to think carefully and examine the evidence around them, considering what factors promote success and what factors impede it. This will include consideration of factors such as group versus individual work, whether the gender of the therapist has any impact, what is most useful for single parents, whether programmes need to be altered to met the needs of specific groups, e.g. low-income families, different ethnic groups. A useful starting point for such research is Taylor and Biglan's 1998 literature review.

Two programmes with strong evidence are the Webster Stratton Incredible Years programme (Webster Stratton 1992, 1998) and the Triple P Positive Parenting Programme (Sanders *et al.* 2000). These programmes share a number of features:

- *Teaching practical strategies to building a positive parent child relationship.* The main focus is *child-led play* – showing parents how to play with their child in a way that encourages the child to develop imaginative/symbolic play and helps the parent to learn about their child and how they see themselves and their world. It's also meant to be a fun time, where the child has the chance to make the rules and decide how things are going to happen. This is especially important for children with ADHD, when a lot of emphasis is on developing structured routines with clear rules and expectations. Unless this is balanced with regular episodes of child-led play the children often struggle to know what to do with unstructured times, e.g. going to play at a friend's house. Helping children develop the capacity for symbolic play is also important in the later development of coping strategies and self-expression (Wilson *et al.* 1992).
- *Clear rules and rewards for compliance.* Parents are asked to make a list of behaviours they would like to see more of (rather than all the things they wish the child didn't do) and work out reward systems around these. For example, children who struggle to do as they are asked might have a chart that gives them a point every time they do as they are asked (first time). Depending on the age of child and stage of development, rewards may be given straight away (this would be appropriate with a 3-year-old) and may take the form of stickers or verbal praise. Older children may be able to collect points towards a reward. Children are usually very good at thinking of things they would like to work towards and it is useful for them to become part of the behaviour management programme (teaching self-monitoring and self-evaluation). The key factors when using this kind of programme is the rewards must be achievable (never more than a week to achieve even in middle childhood) and realistic, both in terms of budget and time.
- Parents are taught behaviour management strategies such as ignoring and distraction for 'low-level' behaviour difficulties (e.g. whining, baby talk).

- Parents are encouraged to reduce the number of commands they give their children and to phrase them in a clear, unambiguous way.
- Clear sanctions are put in place for severe, persistent misbehaviour, e.g. violence. Both programmes advocate the use of time out rather than shouting or smacking as being more effective in helping children to develop more appropriate behaviour.

Both programmes are most effective when run as groups (typically 2 hours once a week for 3–6 months) but the principles can form the basis of work with individual parents. The triple P programme was shown to be particularly effective in improving the child's behaviour, decreasing symptoms of ADHD and changing parental attitudes towards the child when used with younger children who had recently been diagnosed with ADHD (Pelham *et al.* 1988). This programme uses cognitive behavioural approaches, which have been shown to be particularly effective with children with ADHD (Pistermann *et al.* 1989).

Individual work with the child

One of the major difficulties for children with ADHD is the ability to self-regulate – by this I mean the ability to tune into themselves and how they are feeling, and to formulate a response to the situation based on this information and an assessment of the environment, which may include another person and how they might be feeling. Using the detailed steps researched by attachment theorists, neurobiologists and neurophysiologists it is possible for the occupational therapist to plan a remedial programme of work with the child and the parent, replicating the pattern of normal development but amplifying and consolidating areas of particular need.

Theory underpinning the intervention

There is general agreement among attachment theorists and neuroscientists that, in normal development, a secure attachment relationship is vital in the child developing the ability to modulate and regulate their levels of arousal. Successful completion of this process is dependent on both the infant expressing need and the parent consistently and repeatedly meeting those needs.

Attachment theorists (such as Bowlby, Ainsworth, Sroufe, Stevenson-Hinde, Stern) bring together strands of biology, neurophysiology and psychoanalysis and stress the importance of the early bond formed between the mother (or main caregiver) and the child. This is a complex process, which continues to be the subject of much research (Murray and Andrews 2000, Trevarthin 2001). There is general consensus that this process involves a matching of the mother to the child in which the mother's responsiveness to the infant signals and her ability to respond appropriately and meet their physical and emotional aspects determine the quality of the attachment relationship (Lieberman and Pawl (1990), Ainsworth (1991), McCluskey (2005)). Neurophysiologists describe the 'synchronised interactions' between caregiver and child (Kopp 1982, Penman *et al.* 1983). Children with ADHD often struggle to express their needs in a way that makes it easy for the caregiver to understand and respond to them and so the cycle of attachment is often incomplete.

Van der Kolk and Fisler (1994) discuss the importance of a secure attachment relationship if the child is to develop the ability to modulate physiological arousal. If the infant has not had the experience of a secure attachment relationship they suggest that the child will struggle to understand and process their own feelings. They link this to the child's impaired ability to use symbolism or differentiate and express their feelings verbally. Again this is of relevance when working with children with ADHD in planning a treatment programme to remediate some of these gaps.

What attachment theorists have observed and described in terms of human relationships, neurobiologists have looked at as structural changes in the developing brain. Schore (1999) emphasises the importance of the secure attachment in forming a neurological foundation for the subsequent development of the right hemispheric orbitofrontal cortex which becomes the control centre for the regulation and modulation of levels of arousal as well as the expression of emotion, development of empathy and development of peer group relationships. He links Bowlby's description of a process of development, e.g. increasing attachment behaviours between 7 and 15 months with the period of critical myelination and maturation of rapidly developing limbic and cortical association areas (Schore 2000). Rabinowicz (1979) (cited in Schore 2000) describes limbic areas of the human cortex showing anatomical maturation at 15 months. Heineman (1998) also studied the formation of neurobiological pathways in the frontal and parietal lobes, studying the effects of different styles of attachment on their formation.

It is important to note that although much research and writing on attachment theory concentrates on the period of early infancy, attachment patterns established during infancy are not immovable, and our patterns of attachment relationships are honed and changed throughout our lives according to our experiences. In particular, there is evidence that early attachment patterns are amenable to change in the context of a therapeutic relationship (e.g. van Ijzendoorn *et al.* 1994, Cicchetti *et al.* 1999, Howe and Fearnley 1999).

Practical Application – Feelingometers and Feeling Catchers – helping children to develop an internal working model for managing and regulating levels of arousal

The author has developed a three-part treatment programme for the child and parent using the theoretical frameworks outlined above, following and replicating this pattern of normal attachment behaviour. The basic principle is to follow the path of the development of a secure attachment relationship, the mother beginning as the more active interactant in the process, the child following her lead and gradually becoming competent and confident in their experiencing and expressing of their emotional world.

The first part of the programme involves the therapist establishing a relationship with the child and beginning the process of helping them name and describe feelings. In the second part the parent tries to notice and to 'catch' the child having certain feelings and records these, noticing the circumstances surrounding the feeling and gradually helping the child to tune into their own emotional world. The third part concentrates on the behaviour that follows the feeling, and uses the parent–child interaction to make links between feelings and subsequent/consequent behaviour. This is divided into ways of managing the feelings that were useful and ways of managing the feelings that led to difficulties. From here strategies are developed for expressing and managing more difficult feelings as well as consideration of any environmental changes or changes in parenting style that could facilitate the child's process of change. This final part of the process draws on the research and evidence for the efficacy of cognitive, behavioural and psychosocial interventions for children with ADHD (Abikoff 1991, Pelham *et al.* 1999).

Stage 1 – naming the feelings

Stage 1 involves a number of weekly sessions with the child. During this stage, the therapist tries to establish an effective relationship with the child, by acknowledging the difficulties in recognising and managing feelings. The purpose of the therapy is emphasised, generally this is explained as a way of helping them recognise, name and manage their feelings using a range of different activities.

This is a directive therapy. Consequently the therapist has prepared the session for the child and leads the child into the work. In the initial sessions the therapist helps the child to think of as many words as they can for feelings. These are written on a big piece of paper. It is important at this stage not to make links between these feelings and the child, but just to get as big a list as possible of feeling words. This is because at this stage of therapy children are often confused or perplexed by feeling words or think that some are 'bad' feelings that they should not be talking about. Children often find it easier of think of feeling words like sad and angry but struggle to think of words like proud, excited or hardworking. It doesn't matter if it is the therapist or the child who suggests words for feelings, as long as there is a selection of feelings on the page.

The next step is to ask the child to circle any words that they might have felt at any time. It seems important to phrase the request like this, especially if the child finds it difficult to recognise or talk about feelings – it allows them to remain one step removed from the process.

The child is then asked to grade the feelings according to how easy or difficult they are to recognise, express or manage. It is important to avoid pejorative terms like good and bad feelings – the message that the therapist is trying to convey is that there is nothing inherently good or bad about any feelings, but that some are trickier to recognise and manage than others. The child (or therapist) then draws some sort of a measuring instrument – this may be as simple as a straight line on the paper or may be more complex like a speedometer – which is then divided up into three areas: an area for feelings that are easy to feel or think about, one for feelings that are trickier to feel or think about and an 'in between' area. The therapist then helps the child to decide where on this spectrum to place the different feeling words that they have identified and cut them out and stick them on appropriately.

The next part of this stage of therapy is to help children to think about individual feelings. This may involve painting/art work, e.g. if this piece of paper was the feeling lonely, what would it look like, what sort of shape would it be, would it be one colour or lots of different colours, would it take up the whole paper or just be a small part of the paper? The important part of this process is not the finished picture but the child beginning to try to 'get inside' the different feelings and portray them in some way. The aim is to help the child to become accustomed to talking and thinking about feelings. This helps them to gain some mastery over the feelings, developing a sense that they may be able to manage feelings that at the time feel very out of control.

Although it is important to go with the child's interpretation of a feeling it is also important to correct the child if they are using the wrong word for a feeling, e.g. if a child thinks that the feeling word to describe when you're feeling really good because you've tried really hard and succeeded at something is 'envious', it would be important to talk to them about the word 'proud', as that is the word that most people use to describe that feeling.

For some children, this part of the therapy is too abstract, they struggle to imagine what feelings might look like. Something more concrete may be helpful – such as drawing the outline of a figure and asking them to colour where in their body they feel that feeling.

Stage 2 – 'Feeling Catchers' – catching the feelings

Once a common language has been established for feelings and there is some differentiation between feelings that are easier or harder to feel and to express, it is time to move on to the next stage of therapy. The aim of the 'feeling catcher' stage of therapy is to help the parent and child notice what and how they are feeling in everyday situations. This begins, as in the early attachment relationship, by helping the mother tune into how the child is feeling at specific points in the day. From here, therapy moves to helping the child consider the accuracy of the mother's surmising, allowing them to work together on 'catching' feelings as they happen in day-to-day life. Eventually this allows for consideration of how the child manages these feelings, differentiating between helpful and unhelpful strategies, allowing the development of appropriate ways of managing and expressing feelings. This mirrors the first stage of the process of attunement in the normal attachment process, where the mother is the more active interactant, trying to decipher the signals of the infant and understand the underlying feelings. Keeping

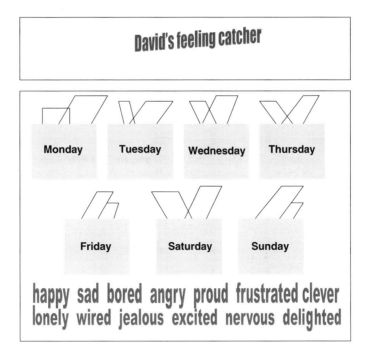

Figure 2.1 David's feeling catcher.

the emphasis on underlying feelings also helps break the cycle of parents constantly focusing on the child's behaviour. It is perhaps best to illustrate this process with an example.

David is an 8-year-old boy who had been excluded from school because of his difficult behaviour. He had been diagnosed with ADHD and as being on the autistic spectrum. At home there were constant rows and fights between David and his younger sibling and mother was frequently bruised and hurt in these encounters. David's 'feelingometer' was fairly sparse, with only brave and delighted at the easier to manage end of the spectrum and guilty, lonely, cross and angry at the difficult to manage end.

For the first session I made a feeling catcher (Figure 2.1) with a couple of pockets for each day of the week. It is important to make the charts look interesting and appealing – I use brightly coloured paper or card, different ways of writing, to keep it interesting and stop it looking too much like homework from school.

I asked David and his mother to sit down and think of a couple of things that had happened that day, and for mum to write down the event and also a couple of feeling words that she thought might match how David had been feeling. At this stage, the mother and child are not asked to make any comments about what has happened or mother's thoughts, but simply to go through the exercise and bring it the next week to therapy.

For David and his mother, the first week brought a good range of feelings: proud and brave for resisting his sister's attempts to goad him into a fight, loved

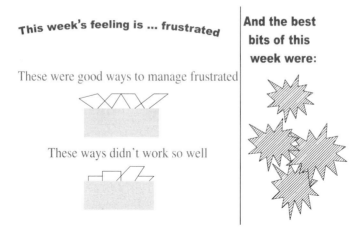

Figure 2.2 Evaluation of feelings management.

and delighted at helping granny make a chocolate cake, angry and upset when being told off for breaking a chair and frustrated when his magazine was out of stock at the local shops. We spent the first 15 minutes of the second session opening the pockets of the feeling catcher, and David obviously enjoyed the reflection and reviewing of the week, particularly the parts where mum was full of praise for the way that he had handled himself in tricky situations.

Keeping the emphasis on underlying feelings also helps breaking the cycle of parents constantly complaining about the child's behaviour, making this the only thing that the child often hears when they are brought to the clinic. From here things progress to refining the feeling catcher and focusing on three or four feelings for the next week. Figure 2.2 shows what a typical feeling catcher from this stage of therapy might look like.

Stage 3 – Making links between feelings and behaviour and modifying the behaviour

At this stage the emphasis changes from merely 'catching' the feelings to thinking about how the child managed those feelings. The focus each week is now on one specific feeling that the parent and child have agreed often leads to difficulties and the task is not only to catch that feeling but also to analyse what happened next. Feeling catchers are expanded to include paper pockets for ways of managing the feeling that worked well and pockets for ways of managing the feeling that didn't work so well. In addition, there is a section on the chart (I usually make it a gold cup or some sort of trophy that is meaningful to the child) for recording things that have gone very well for the child, or examples of times that they managed other difficult feelings well. This section is particularly important in continuing to develop the child's self-esteem and sense of themselves when the emphasis of the sessions moves on to more difficult feelings.

It is important that the feelings chosen for each week are feelings that are difficult for the child but manageable. The child must be able to succeed at each stage of the process and feelings to be caught must be graded appropriately. It may be appropriate at this stage of therapy to lengthen the gaps between sessions, up to a maximum of every four weeks. This may be graded according to the degree of engagement and confidence of the parent. Therapy continues until the child has become competent in managing and expressing even the most difficult feelings.

Adaptations to the model

The feeling catcher part of the therapy can be adapted in many ways to meet the needs of both child and parent. It is important to analyse any difficulties that the parent and child may be having with the week's homework and not necessarily to assume that the difficulties lie with the child.

Some of the times when in my experience this has not been an effective technique is when the parent has been unable to be a part of the therapy. This has sometimes been because they are so angry with the child for the anguish the child has caused that they are unable to be balanced in their view of the things that the child does well and the things that the child is struggling with. It can sometimes be effective to spend time helping the parent move from this position, but again this can be difficult.

There have also been times when it has been useful to transfer the basic principle of the feeling catcher into the classroom situation. This has been particularly useful when schools have been struggling to notice the triggers to a child's behaviour or are struggling to see when a child is doing well.

Work with school

Education about ADHD is of prime importance (Royal College of Psychiatrists have produced useful fact sheets for parents and teachers of children with ADHD, and these are available from their website (www.rcpsych.ac.uk)). In addition there is evidence from Southampton Child and Mental Health Services (CAMHS) resources that cognitive, behavioural and psychosocial strategies are useful in improving performance in the classroom and in building peer group relationships (Workman and Dickinson 1979, Zentall and Leib 1985, DuPaul and Eckert 1997).

░ Theory into practice 6 ░

Work was done with Gavin's class teacher about changing the environment of the classroom to facilitate Gavin's learning and overall success. These things included:

░ Moving Gavin's seat to the group of children who sat closest to the teacher. Teachers sometimes put disruptive children at the back of the classroom to minimise the effects of their disruption on the rest of the class. This is not appropriate for children with ADHD who need to be sitting close to the teacher so that they can be prompted and brought back on task regularly.

▪ Setting up different areas in the classroom for quiet working – Gavin's teacher quickly realised that the ideal environment for Gavin was a quiet, unstimulating one and devised a simple but effective and non-stigmatising system to make this happen. Over a period of days she told the class about a special new workstation that was going to be just around the corner from the main hub of the class. Each day children could earn points to allow them to go into this special zone. The children were all excited at the thought of this and worked really hard to be allowed to go to this special spot in the class. The teacher gave Gavin a regular morning job that he enjoyed (taking the register along to the secretary) which allowed him to earn points for being helpful and co-operative and so earn a place in the work station. There were never more than three people there at a time and the learning assistant worked with them. This was a clever and creative way of allowing Gavin to succeed without it seeming like a punishment – go and work in the cloakroom.

▪ Encouraging the teacher to vary her presentation, interspersing it with physical activities and varying the tone and style of presentation to keep interest levels high.

▪ Regular prompts by the teacher when it was really important for Gavin to listen. Encouraging her to start saying things like 'And this is the really important thing you need to know' or 'Here's the crucial piece of information'.

▪ Clear, simple goals for playtime worked out with the lunchtime and playtime supervisors.

For other children and teachers the following have been found to be useful when working with children with ADHD.

▪ *Closed plan classrooms* are easier because they are generally quieter and have fewer distractions (Green and Chee 1994).

▪ *Helping the child to develop clear routines.* For example, the teacher writing up a plan of the day on the board and encouraging practical activity analysis – breaking tasks down into manageable stages and considering the impact of the environment.

▪ *Clear, concise, stepped instructions.*

Other interventions that can be useful for schools include:

▪ *Using sensory integration techniques to help the child regulate their physiological arousal.* Some programmes such as the Alert (Williams and Shellenberger 1992) approach are also useful in helping children tune into their level of physiological arousal and developing strategies to manage this. This programme would seem to be more widely used by paediatric occupational therapists than CAMHS occupational therapists but there could be useful collaboration, linking areas of emotional and physiological arousal. This is an area that will benefit from further research.

▪ *Whole-school approaches to teach children skills in communication and conflict resolution.* A particularly good example of this is the Second Step programme (Committee for Children 2002), a research-based programme for school-age children which uses weekly classroom-based lessons to teach communication skills which are then practised and reinforced throughout the day in the classroom and around school. There are three modules per year – empathy training (learning to tune into feelings and beginning to imagine what it might be like to be someone else), impulse control and anger management. The lessons give clear structures which teach children how to calm down and ways to resolve conflicts and differences which are fair and safe. One advantage of the Second Step programme is that it is skills based and classroom led. This gives the teacher the opportunity to model and reinforce the skills throughout the school day. Non-teaching staff are also trained in the techniques and so these are also used in the playground and other areas around school. This consistency of highly structured approach is particularly helpful for children with ADHD and can easily be transferred to the home. (An important part of the programme is the home–school liaison, and parents are given information about the skills and how they are taught.)

Evaluation

It is useful to refer back to the assessment phase of treatment when considering evaluation and to re-test the child using the same standardised assessments (e.g. Conners, Achenbach). Other interventions in the package of treatment may be standardised and have their own battery of pre- and post-intervention measures, e.g. the Webster Stratton parent training programme measures parental stress as well as the child's level of difficulty before and after treatment. The Walker and McConnell scale (1995) of emotional competence and school adjustment is useful in measuring the child's level of understanding of feelings and their ability to change their behaviour in response to this information within the school setting. It is completed by the class teacher. Again, it is designed to be used before and after an intervention.

Closing remarks

ADHD is a complex condition that can lead to serious long-term difficulties for children and young people if left untreated. As has been discussed, treatment is most effective if it can be multimodal, delivered by a multi-disciplinary team and tailored to meet the needs of the individual child and family. It is sometimes difficult not to be overwhelmed by the enormity of the task in treating these children, who often think that they are stupid and no good, and their families, who may have suffered years of blame and rejection because of their child's behaviour. It is crucial to have a clear idea of the contribution of the occupational therapist to the treatment team.

Occupational therapists' expertise in working with children to develop self-regulation, both emotional and physiological, and their strength in analysing tasks of daily living (looking at the influences of the environment as well as the strengths and difficulties of the individual) mean that they are important members of the treatment team. Treatment must encompass all areas of the child's life: play, leisure, school, family life and friendships.

There is, as yet, little empirical evidence of the efficacy of the occupational therapy intervention for children with ADHD. In building the evidence for working with children with ADHD it is important to look at the theories of normal development and recent research in psychology, psychoanalysis, neuro-physiology and neurobiology. Addressing the question of how during normal development children develop the capacity to regulate and modulate their levels of physical and emotional arousal can form a foundation for work with children with ADHD and can be combined with research and literature on approaches that are successful for children with ADHD and their families. There is a real need for more research, especially around the interventions used by occupational therapists working with children with ADHD that incorporate the different approaches of paediatric and child and adolescent mental health occupational therapy.

References

Abikoff, H. (1991) Cognitive training with children with ADHD: Less to it than meets the eye. *Journal Of Learning Disabilities.* **24**: 205–9.

Achenbach, T.M. (1991) *Manual For The Child Behaviour Checklist/4–18 and 1991 Profile.* Burlington: University of Vermont, Department of Psychiatry.

Ainsworth, M. (1991) Attachment and other affectional bonds across the life cycle. In: Parkes, C.M., Stevenson–Hinde, J. and Marris, P. (eds) *Attachment Across The Life Cycle.* London: Routledge.

APA (1994) *Diagnostic and Statistical Manual of Mental Disorders – Fourth Edition (DSM-IV).* Washington DC: American Psychiatric Association.

Barkley, R.A. (1991) The ecological validity of laboratory and analogue assessment methods of ADHD. *Journal of Abnormal Child Psychology.* **19**: 149–78.

Bramble, D. (2003) Annotation; the use of psychotropic medication in children: a British view. *Journal of Child Psychology and Psychiatry.* **44**: 169–79.

Chu, S. (2003) Occupational therapy for children with attention deficit hyperactivity disorder: a survey of the level of involvement and training needs of therapists. *British Journal Of Occupational Therapy.* **66**(5): 209–18.

Cicchetti, D., Toth, S. and Rogosch, F. (1999) The efficacy of toddler parent psychotherapy to increase attachment security in offspring of depressed mothers. *Attachment and Human Development.* **1**: 34–66.

Committee For Children (2002) *Second Step: A Violence Prevention Curriculum.* Seattle, WA: Committee For Children. Website: www.cfchildren.org

Conners, C.K. (1989) *Conners Rating Scale Manual.* New York: Multi-Health Systems. Includes the parents and teachers rating scales.

Dumas, J. (1989) Treating antisocial behaviour in children: child and family approaches. *Clinical Psychology Review.* **9**: 197–222.

DuPaul, G. and Eckert, T.L. (1997) The effects of school-based interventions for attention deficit hyperactivity disorder: a meta analysis. *School Psychology Review.* **23**: 5–27.

Fergusson, D.M., Horwood, L.J. and Lloyd, M. (1991) Confirmatory factor models of attention deficit and conduct disorder. *Journal of Child Psychology and Psychiatry.* **21**: 257–74.

Gillberg, C., Meander, H., von Knorring, A., Janols, L., Thernlund, G., Heaggloef, B., Eideval-Wallin, L., Gustaffson, P. and Kopp, S. (1997) Long term stimulant treatment of children with ADHD symptoms – a randomised, double blind, placebo-controlled study. *Archives of General Psychiatry*. **54**: 857–64.

Gillberg, C., Gillberg, I.C., Rasmussen, P., Kadesjo, B., Soderstrom, H., Rastam, M., Johnson, M., Rothenberg, A. and Nicklasson, L. (2004) Co-existing disorders in ADHD: Implications for diagnosis and intervention. *European Child and Adolescent Psychiatry*. **13**(Suppl.): 180–92.

Green, C. and Chee, K. (1994) *Understanding ADHD. The Definitive Guide to Attention Deficit Hyperactivity Disorder*. New York: Fawcett.

Heineman, T. (1998) *The Abused Child: Psychodynamic Understanding and Treatment*. New York: The Guilford Press.

Horn, W., Ialongo, N., Greenberg, G., Packard, T. and Smith Winberry, C. (1990) Additive effects of behavioural parent training and self-control therapy with ADHD children. *Journal of Clinical Child Psychology*. **19**: 98–110.

Horn, W., Ialongo, N., Greenberg, G., Pascoe, J., Lopez, M., Wagner, A. and Puttler, L. (1991) Additive effects of psychostimulants, parent training and self-control therapy with ADHD children: a 9 month follow up. *Journal of the American Academy of Child and Adolescent Psychiatry*. **32**: 182–9.

Howe, D. and Fearnley, S. (1999) Disorders of attachment and attachment therapy. *Adoption and Fostering*. **23**: 19–29.

Jennings, S. (ed.) (1995) *Dramatherapy with Children and Adolescents*. London: Routledge.

Jensen, P. (2002) Longer term effects of stimulant medication for attention deficit hyperactivity disorder. *Journal Of Attentional Disorders*. **6**(Suppl.1): 45–56.

Kadzin, A. (1991) *Conduct Disorders in Childhood and Adolescence*. Thousand Oaks, CA: Sage Publications.

Klein, R. and Menuzza, S. (1991) Long term outcomes of hyperactive children. *Journal of The American Academy of Child and Adolescent Psychiatry*. **30**: 383–7.

Knapp, P. and Deluty, R. (1989) Relative effectiveness of two behavioural parent training programmes. *Journal of Clinical Child Psychology*. **18**: 314–22.

Kopp, C. (1982) Antecedents of self regulation: a developmental perspective. *Developmental Psychology*. **18**: 199–214.

Lieberman, A. and Pawl, J. (1990) Disorders of attachment and secure base behaviour in the second year of life. In: Greenberg, M., Cicchetti, D. and Cummings, E. (eds) *Attachment In the Pre-school Years*. London: University of Chicago Press.

Mangeot, S., Miller, L., McGrathe-Clarke, J., Hagerman, R. and Goldson, E. (2001) Sensory modulation dysfunction in children with attention deficit hyperactivity disorder. *Developmental Medicine and Childhood Neurology*. **43**: 399–406.

McCluskey, U. (2005) *A Theory of Care Giving in Adult Life: Developing and Measuring the Concept of Goal Corrective Empathic Attunement*. London: Karnac Books.

Murray, L. and Andrews, L. (2000) *The Social Baby*. Richmond, UK: Children's Project Publishing.

NICE (2000) *Guidance on the Use of Methylphenidate (Ritalin, Equasym) for Attention Deficit/Hyperactivity Disorder in Childhood*. Technology Appraisal Guidance No. 13. London: National Institute of Clinical Excellence.

Pelham, W.E., Wheeler, T. and Chronsis, A. (1988) Behaviour intervention in attention deficit/ hyperactivity disorder. In: Quay, H. and Hogan, G. (eds) *Handbook of Disruptive Disorders*. New York: Kluwer Academic/Plenium.

Pelham, W.E., Wheeler, T. and Chronis, A. (1999) Empirically supported psychosocial treatments for attention deficit hyperactivity disorder. *Journal of Clinical Child Psychology.* **27**: 190–205.

Penman, R., Mearns, R. and Milgrom-Friedman, J. (1983) Synchronicity in mother–infant interaction: a possible neurophysiological base. *British Journal of Medical Psychology.* **56**: 1–7.

Pisterman, S., McGrath, P., Firestone, P. and Goodman, J. (1989) Outcome of parent-mediated treatment of preschoolers with attention deficit disorder with hyperactivity. *Journal of Consulting and Clinical Psychology.* **57**: 628–35.

Rabinowicz, T. (1979) The differentiate maturation of the human cerebral cortex. In: Falkner, F. and Tanner, J. (eds) *Human Growth Vol. 3 Neurobiology and Nutrition*. New York: Plenum Press, pp. 223–355.

Royal College of Psychiatrists (1999) Mental Health and Growing Up Factsheet no. 5. *Attention Deficit Problems and Hyperactivity.*

Sanders, M., Markie Dodds, C. and Turner, K. (2000) *Every Parent's Survival Guide: Triple P – Positive Parenting Programme*. Milton, Queensland: Triple P International Pty Ltd. Website: www.triplep.net

Schore, A. (1999) *Affect Regulation and the Development of the Self: The Neurobiology of Emotional Development*. Mahwah, NJ: Lawrence Erbaum.

Schore, A. (2000) Attachment and the regulation of the right brain. *Attachment and Human Development.* **2**: 23–47.

Semud-Clikeman, M., Biederman, J. and Sprich-Buckminster, D. (1992) Comorbidity between ADHD and learning disability: a review and report of clinically referred sample. *Journal of the American Academy of Child and Adolescent Psychiatry.* **31**: 439–88.

Sergeant, J.A., Geurts, H. and Oosterland, J. (2002) How specific is a deficit of executive functioning for attention deficit hyperactivity disorder? *Behaviour and Brain Research.* **130**: 3–28.

SIGN (2001) *Attention Deficit Hyperkinetic Disorder in Children And Young People*. SIGN guideline no 52. Edinburgh: Scottish Intercollegiate Guidelines Network.

Taylor, E., Dopfner, M., Sergeant, J., Asherton, P., Banaschewski, T., Buitelaar, T., Coghill, D., Danckaerts, M., Rothenberger, A., Sonuga-Barke, E., Steinhausen, H. and Zuddas, A. (2004) European clinical guidelines for hyperkinetic disorder – first upgrade. *European Child and Adolescent Psychiatry.* **13**: Suppl. 1.

Taylor, T. and Biglan, A. (1998) Behavioural family interventions for improving child rearing: a review of the literature for clinicians and policy makers. *Clinical Child and Family Psychology.* **1**: 41–60.

Trevarthin, C. (2001) The neurobiology of early communication: intersubjective regulations in human brain development. In: Kalverboer, A.F. and Gramsbergen, A. (eds). *Handbook on Brain and Behavior in Human Development*. Dodrecht, the Netherlands: Kluwer, pp. 841–82.

Van der Kolk, B. and Fisler, R. (1994) Child abuse and neglect and the loss of self regulation. *Bulletin of the Menninger Clinic.* **58**: 145–69.

Van Ijzendoorn, M., Juffer, F. and Duyvesteyn, M. (1994) Breaking the cycle of insecure attachment: a review of the effects of maternal sensitivity on infant security. *Journal of Child Psychology and Psychology* **36**: 225–48.

Walker, H. and McConnell, S. (1995) *Scale of Social Competence and School Adjustment, Elementary Version: Users Manual*. San Diego, CA: Singular Publishing Group Inc.

Webster Stratton, C. (1992) *The incredible Years: A Trouble Shooting Guide for Parents of Children Aged 3–8*. Ontario: Umbrella Press.

Webster Stratton, C. and Taylor, T. (1998) Adopting and implementing empirically supported interventions: a recipe for success. In: Buchanan, A. (ed.) *Parenting, Schooling and Children's Behaviour – Interdisciplinary Approaches*. Hampshire: Ashgate Publishing.

Wenar, C. (1994) *Developmental Psychopathology from Infancy through Adolescence*. New York: McGraw Hill.

West, J. (1996) *Child Centred Play Therapy*. London: Arnold.

Whalen, C. (1989) Attention deficit and hyperactivity disorders. In: Ollendick, T. and Hersen, M. (eds) *Handbook of Childhood Psychopathology*. New York: Plenum, pp. 131–69.

Williams, M. and Shellenberger, S. (1992) *An Introduction to 'How Does Your Engine Run?' The Alert Programme for Self Regulation*. Albuquerque, NM: Therapy Works.

Wilson, K., Kendrick, P. and Ryan, V. (1992) *Play Therapy; A Non Directive Approach for Children and Adolescents*. London: Baillière Tindall.

Workman, E. and Dickinson, D. (1979) The use of covert positive reinforcement in the treatment of the hyperactive child: an empirical case study. *Journal of School Psychology*. **17**: 67–73.

Zentall, S. and Leib, S. (1985) Structured tasks: effects on activity and performance of hyperactive and comparison children. *Journal of Educational Research*. **79**: 91–5.

3: Enhancing self-efficacy in managing major depression

Gill Richmond

This chapter explores developments in cognitive-behavioural therapy (CBT) that are relevant for evidence-based, psychosocial occupational therapy practice. Elements of CBT for depression will be discussed. Yerxa (2000) highlights the need for occupational therapists to follow her lead and become detectives in tracking down relevant areas of research to inform practice, provided they are consistent with the values held by occupational therapists.

The impact of depression

Depression is a leading cause of disability throughout the world, severely disrupting social and occupational functioning and creating an increased risk of completed suicide (Doris *et al.* 1999). A report by Lord Layard (2004) highlights the need to target treatment at those whose depression prevents them from being able to function in their usual lives. Current statistics show that 20% of people with depression remain unwell two years after diagnosis, and relapse is a common feature of depression (National Institute for Clinical Excellence (NICE) 2004). Occupational therapists have a major role to play in alleviating the deprived occupational and social experience associated with depression, and in the prevention of further episodes.

The intention of this chapter is to raise awareness and encourage debate on the evidence for strategies that may enhance the client's self-efficacy in managing depression (Bandura 1997). Occupational therapists need to judge how far these strategies lead to enhanced well-being, improved function and quality of life, and how far they protect against the impact of low mood on competence and self-identity (Mee *et al.* 2004).

This chapter will help you to explore the relevance of the 'landmark studies of efficacy' for the treatment of depression (Roth and Fonaghy 2005). Links are made with current recommendations on the management of working age adults with depression in primary and secondary care (NICE 2004). Selected, applied examples of CBT indicate how occupational therapy can be underpinned by a specific evidence-based treatment model. Illustrations are drawn from an anonymised case example reflecting Mira's experience of treatment for a major depressive episode (*Diagnostic and Statistical Manual of Mental Disorders* (DSM-IV), American Psychiatric Association 2000). This is classified as moderate to severe according to the International Classification of Diseases (ICD)-10 criteria (World Health Organization (WHO) 1992). A complete case study is not provided.

CBT is defined as a self-help model (Blenkiron 1999). It can be offered on an individual, group or self-help basis. In individual psychotherapy it has a directive, highly structured, time-limited approach applied in the context of an active and collaborative therapeutic relationship (Beck *et al.* 1979). The theoretical rationale for the model was originally proposed by Beck (1967, 1976), who stated that a person's mood, experience and behaviour are mainly influenced by specific thoughts and beliefs. This theory has also led to the development of disorder-specific models of emotional disorders of which the first was depression (Beck *et al.* 1979).

CBT has been the most rigorously researched psychological treatment for unipolar depression without psychotic features (NICE 2004). Emphasis has been placed on validating theoretical concepts and outcomes of cognitive behavioural treatment (Tarrier and Calam 2002). In spite of this rigor it is important to apply general principles when analysing the strengths and limitations of each study. Westen and Morrison (2001) highlight four key questions to help weigh the accuracy and utility of conclusions drawn from empirical studies examining outcomes of treatment for depression.

- What is meant by efficacy in this study?
- Do treatment responses refer to initial effects or to sustained effects?
- What distinction is made between disorder-specific treatment versus treatment of states?
- Has the treatment been invalidated by the findings of research or has it been empirically tested to date?

Treatment protocols using CBT have been found to be particularly helpful under the following circumstances: when antidepressant medication regimens may be unsuitable owing to a high risk of suicide through overdose; noncompliance with medication; side-effects or poor tolerance; additional medication for other issues, which interact adversely with psychotropic medication; co-morbid psychiatric disorders such as personality disorders or substance misuse; or for clients who do not improve on medication (Scott 1996).

Paykel (2002) reviewed outcomes of treatment for depression where adverse effects were noted in spite of the use of modern anti-depressants. This review draws attention to the slow rate in the return of social functioning compared with reduction in depressive symptoms. Particular difficulties were noted in adaptation to work-related roles. This suggests that occupational therapists need to focus on identifying additional criterion-based occupational and social markers to track and evaluate the efficacy of treatment gains beyond symptom reduction. Focusing on treatment strategies specifically designed to enhance social and occupational functioning may mitigate against recurrence and relapse. More research is required to support or dispute this assertion. There is more discussion on the evidence base for cognitive behavioural interventions later in the chapter.

Further elements which need to be considered are the limiting factors and problems arising from current descriptions and diagnostic criteria for depression (NICE 2004). This may affect the value of research and creates difficulties in planning interventions. To explore these points further you may wish to examine the current criteria for major depressive disorder described in *Diagnostic and Statistical Manual of Mental Disorders* (DSM-IV) (APA 2000).

Check through the diagnostic criteria and consider the following questions related to the case example illustrated in this chapter. How helpful are the current diagnostic criteria in helping us to understand:

- The personal experience of depression?
- The causes of the depression for this person?
- What form of intervention is likely to be most useful?
- The impact on occupational and social performance?

In addition to exploring the strengths and limitations of diagnostic criteria the following example provides an opportunity to explore the utility of CBT in enhancing social and occupational function and alleviating the symptoms of depression. You may wish to consider how you would develop the therapeutic relationship and help to establish a collaborative and culturally sensitive working relationship as Mira is socialised into the process of therapy. Acting against any indication of shame and stigma is a key task at this stage (Gilbert *et al.* 2004). Psycho-educational material tailored to Mira's needs would be provided to help normalise her experience of depression and answer any queries such as how to use anti-depressant medication effectively. Pseudonyms have been used throughout and details changed to preserve anonymity.

Mohanbir Kaur (pseudonym) was referred by her general practitioner to a community mental health team. The referral letter stated that she was a 34-year-old woman recovering from her third depressive episode. She was married with two children aged 3 and 9 years.

Mohanbir preferred to be called Mira. The narrative of her experience of depression was collected over three sessions. Mira was an active member of the Sikh faith. Her first language was English. She was born and brought up in a large city in the UK. Her mother had moved to the UK after her father had suddenly died of a 'fever' in India. Although her mother had remarried, Mira remembered her mother appeared unhappy in the marriage. She seemed preoccupied with the loss of her first husband and experienced episodes of depression throughout Mira's childhood. From the age of 10 years, Mira was frequently given the responsibility of looking after her four younger siblings.

Mira herself had first experienced depression when she was 19 years old and at university. She was offered six sessions of 'counselling' by the university counsellor and a course of anti-depressants. She found this helpful to deal with the pressure of the course but continued to feel isolated and low periodically. Two years later Mira experienced a further episode of depression which she associated with pressure of final year examinatios in business studies. Anti-depressant medication gradually relieved some of the symptoms but lethargy remained a problem.

Mira linked her current episode of depression to her youngest daughter's diagnosis of epilepsy. Mira said she felt criticised by her mother in law for bringing a 'defective' child into the family. She also reported difficulty adapting to changes in her role at work.

Mira identified difficulties with concentration and 'inability' to cope with everyday tasks such as cooking and caring for the children, and attending to religious duties. Mira was able to manage some of these tasks with prompts from her husband. She described increased lethargy in the morning. She was concerned that her thoughts had slowed down leading her to believe 'I am unable to think'. She had a poor appetite with no enjoyment of food. The key emotions she experienced were 'irritability, sadness and guilt'. Her sleep pattern was disrupted with initial insomnia and early morning wakening. Mira said she felt guilty and distressed every time she looked at sewing material she had intended to make into a dress for her daughter. 'I can't even be bothered to put it away now.' She felt isolated from her friends. Mira disclosed that sometimes when she was alone she had fleeting thoughts of harming herself. She described herself as 'completely helpless and pathetic' for having had these thoughts but was clear that she had never considered acting on them, even when her mood was at its worst. She had been taking Fluoxetine (anti-depressant medication) for six weeks but could not remember the dose. She reported moderate caffeine levels, and had no problems related alcohol or illicit drugs. When she was first seen for initial assessment by the occupational therapist, her mood was beginning to lift and she was able to concentrate for longer periods.

■ How would you assess and monitor the risk of deliberate self-harm; suicide and harm to others; self-neglect; and vulnerability to harm from others?
■ How would you balance risk management with graded risk taking? (See Morgan (2000) for further discussion).
■ What steps could be taken to assess and monitor the well-being of the children?
■ What rationale would you give for seeing Mira at home?
■ Which other assessments would you use?
■ Which other members of the community mental health team could be involved and why?
■ How could cultural competency be ensured during contact with Mira and her family? (See Papadopoulos 2006, Betancourt *et al.* 2002, Sashidharan 2003 for further reading).

Screening for suitability

To decide whether Mira is likely to benefit from CBT, Safran *et al.*'s (1996) ten-item suitability scale is helpful in determining how far this model may address the client's presenting problems and needs. Mira's understanding of the model was elicited, further information was added and a joint discussion established that CBT was likely to be the most acceptable and useful form of therapy for Mira at this point in time.

Mira identified specific self-critical thoughts such as, 'I am a useless wife and mother'. She recognised this as an immediate precursor to her low mood. She responded well to a diagrammatical representation of these links known as the 'initial formulation' (Figure 3.1). Mapping the problem out in the form of a diagram made sense to her and helped her to view the problem as more manageable (Butler 1999).

Mira appeared likely to benefit from CBT for the following reasons:

■ She was willing to look at changes she could make with support.
■ She could describe a relatively discrete problem area.
■ She had demonstrated the ability to identify and work with emotions rather than purely avoiding these.
■ She had responded well to an explanation of the model.

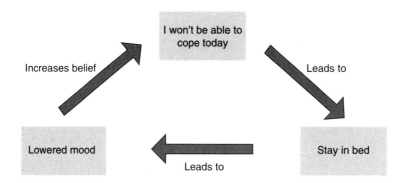

Figure 3.1 Example of an initial formulation.

Mira was able to concentrate quite well in *this* session. Indications of severe but temporary impairment of concentration and memory often seen in depression may indicate that the person requires another approach prior to CBT (Safran *et al.* 1996). See Blenkiron (1999) for a further discussion of suitability of CBT.

The cognitive-behavioural model can be used to target issues that have the potential to reduce the efficacy of the therapy. Clients with personality disorders are likely to require longer-term interventions extending beyond the parameters of the treatment protocol (Vallis *et al.* 2000). Other complicating aspects may be:

▪ past and current evidence of risk issues; relationship difficulties (which could act as a maintaining environmental factor); physical health problems (which could contraindicate certain behavioural experiments) (Safran *et al.* 1996)
▪ low self-esteem; hopelessness; level of anger and irritability; helplessness; use of alcohol; substance abuse; concordance with medication; chronicity of depression; dismissing or minimising the effect/existence of depression; lack of affect (Moore and Garland 2003)
▪ perfectionistic beliefs (Zuroff *et al.* 2000). Therapy may need to be extended beyond its usual timescale to help the client understand and counteract unhelpful aspects of these beliefs (Padesky and Greenberger 1995)

Informed consent for treatment using CBT was gained and the timescale and likely number of sessions was discussed to prepare Mira. NICE guidelines (2004) advocate 16–20 sessions over six to nine months for people experiencing moderate to severe and refractory depression. Mira completed the active phase of therapy in 15 sessions.

Key skills during screening

▪ The first contact needs to include screening for suitability.
▪ Create the first steps in building an effective collaborative relationship.

- Identify potential risks of rupture to the therapeutic relationship.
- Specify the nature of the client's difficulties.
- Clarify initial goals for therapy.
- Agree on the approach to be used/discuss rationale for referral if CBT is not suitable.
- Socialisation to the model is built into this process.
- Therapeutic relationship.

Great emphasis is placed in CBT on 'collaborative empiricism' which means working alongside the client to explore theories generated by the client and therapist on what keeps the problem going and why, testing out the validity of these theories and using a problem-solving approach to help the client develop their ability to make positive changes (Beck *et al.* 1979).

Gilbert (2000) provides a model of depression based on social evolutionary theories which suggests that perceived loss of social rank activates the person's survival mechanisms. Early experiences of social roles that may have been unhelpful, are seen as having the potential to lead to internalisation of self-attacking/shaming cognitive styles. These become more apparent during an episode of depression and can be a major reason for withdrawal from social support. Facilitation *in the client* of a warm and compassionate stance towards his or her own difficulties and needs is advocated. This can be modelled in sessions by the therapist but ultimately needs to be internalised by the client. Particular attention needs to be paid to checking out any perceived criticism in the session by eliciting feedback from the client at regular intervals and whenever there is an indication of increased affect during the session.

Key skills include enhancing motivation and instilling realistic hope (Snyder 2000, Waddington 2002). Increasing value is placed on emotional and interpersonal aspects of CBT which may be combined with the occupational therapist's attention to relational aspects of the therapy known as interactive reasoning (Mattingly 1994).

The definition of the problem acts as a clear statement about the nature of the problem, which the therapist and the client agree to work on. The client's own words are used and jargon is avoided (Williams and Garland 2002, NICE 2004). Mira provided the following problem definition:

> 'I can't work as I get so nervous trying to meet targets. I think I am doing everything wrong. I dwell on these thoughts, ending up feeling confused, tired all the time, and I can't remember anything. I can't concentrate on doing even simple things like cooking properly now. I stay in bed where I feel very low and miserable. I can't shift out of being depressed and believe that I am a failure.'

The problem definition is rated on a scale of 0–8 for intensity of distress generated and the severity of impact on life (Richards and McDonald 1990). Further assessment/outcome measures such as the Beck Depression Inventory (Beck *et al.* 1961) are required to elicit information on the scope and severity of the depression. See Gilbody *et al.* (2001) for a review of measures used in depression and anxiety.

Key skills in collaborative goal setting

- Help the client construct clearly defined, graded, achievable and realistic targets with clear timescales according to the client's priorities.
- Create a first step in helping the client to make effective use of the problem-solving process.

Using the formulation to guide treatment

Therapy is guided by the formulation which Persons (1989) describes as the 'therapist's compass'. This working diagram evolves as client and therapist map aspects of the problem and make hypotheses regarding the interplay between them (Padesky and Greenberger 1995). The impact of the social and occupational environment and context needs to be taken into account (Tarrier and Calam 2002, Whitney *et al.* 2002).

Key skills in using the formulation

- Shared in an overt and collaborative style with clients to assist understanding of links between aspects of the problem and to select, plan and guide intervention.
- Additional information is added to provide flexibility and a comprehensive overview.
- Predict obstacles to applying the treatment plan and facilitate identification of solutions with the client.
- Patterns in behaviour and maintaining factors are mapped out, to help the person understand and predict reactions to specific triggers and experiment with adapting or altering their responses or manipulating the environment (Butler 1999).

The reader may wish to examine the way in which the arrows in Figure 3.2 show links between different aspects of the problem. These maintaining links explain how the depressed mood is triggered, and what keeps it going. They are often described as vicious cycles. Consider how you would use this diagram to work out specific ways to alter or break the links with Mira in treatment. You may wish to add in other single arrows to explain further vicious cycles and consider how these aspects act as triggers or maintaining factors.

Developmental formulation

Roth and Fonaghy (2005) highlight the need for a more detailed classification of depression, which addresses the complexities of the disorder including developmental links to vulnerability factors. In CBT a longitudinal or developmental formulation is intended to assist the client in gaining an understanding of factors which are implicated in the development of depression (Beck *et al.* 1979). Occupational therapists will be familiar with the life history narrative (Kielhofner *et al.*

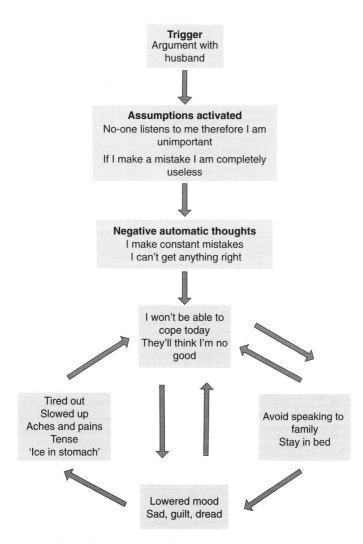

Figure 3.2 Example of a maintenance formulation.

1998). The narrative provides a structure for mapping out specific historical events such as loss or illness which may impact on social and occupational functioning over the person's life span to date. This information can be used as a basis for the developmental formulation. See Gutman and Hayes (2002) for a detailed account of epidemiological factors and theories related to the onset, development and treatment of depression.

Mira felt that the following factors might have been instrumental in leading to her episodes of depression:

▓ Impact of early experiences.
▓ I was expected to take on the role of a parent from the age of about 10 years.

- My mother was unable to care for my needs.
- My stepfather was often angry and irritable, or ignored me unless I was achieving at school.
- These experiences may link with me being careful to avoid upsetting others, feeling I was responsible for the needs of others and that I should ignore my own needs.
- I saw myself as useless and a failure (underlying beliefs).
- Key rules for living (also known as conditional assumptions) may have protected me from feeling completely useless. 'I must try hard to be worth something' 'I must not show my feelings or I will make people angry'.

In Mira's case the critical experiences, which, in theory, activated these rules and beliefs were:

- criticism from mother-in-law;
- changes at work.

The therapist can use questions to help Mira understand how she had responded to these experiences and how they linked with her current experience of depression. In the present situation, Mira's specific beliefs were 'I must not complain about my workload or I will be rejected', and in the context of perceived criticism, 'I must be to blame for my daughter's illness. I am no good as a mother'.

The developmental formulation can be mapped out in diagrammatical form to show the interplay between aspects of the problem (Beck 1976). This leads to a more detailed explanation of why specific triggers such as present criticism contribute more readily to concerns about loss of support and fear of rejection. The detail is crucial to ensure that treatment is targeted effectively. Underlying themes of low self-esteem may be explored to determine specific beliefs held by Mira such as 'I am useless' leading to a decision 'I must put up with unhelpful experiences or I will be rejected'. These may drive rigid judgemental attitudes and evaluations of self (Fennell 1997).

There are questions over how far causality can be established as this will be viewed retrospectively once the person has been diagnosed with depression at a time when autobiographical memory may be affected (Evans *et al.* 1992). For some people, the sheer number of unhelpful early events may seem overwhelming. See Moorey (1996) for a discussion of how the approach can be adjusted to take this into account. The main emphasis in CBT is to help the client gain skills, such as assertion training and problem-solving strategies, to address the here and now with an increased understanding of the personal impact of relevant historical factors.

Style of therapy

Agenda setting is promoted in the Cognitive Therapy Skills–Revised scale (CTS-R) (Blackburn *et al.* 2001). It facilitates attention to specific aspects of the therapy, which include interpersonal aspects. This is particularly helpful in working with complex issues and maintains transparency between therapist and client; mutual agreement on tasks; objective exploration and problem-solving. It promotes structure in the session, which is particularly important in the treatment of depression (Scott *et al.* 1991). The use of structure should enhance a sense of working in partnership. Tasks are negotiated in therapy according to the client's needs and priorities wherever possible. Validation of client goals provides scope to adhere to client-centred principles at the heart of occupational therapy practice (Kusznir and Scott 1999).

Treatment

In this section several aspects of treatment will be explored. Other equally relevant aspects such as the treatment of low self-esteem (Fennell 1997) will not have been covered fully owing to limitations of space. The treatment plan is negotiated collaboratively. It is based on theoretical principles and the model of depression proposed by Beck *et al.* (1979). Moore and Garland (2003) point out difficulties in applying 'standard' models when working with clients such as Mira who experience chronic and persistent symptoms of depression. Emphasis needs to be placed on individualising treatment to attend to areas such as relationship issues that require extra attention.

In the initial phase of therapy, the emphasis was on helping Mira to reduce her symptoms of depression. The aim is to gain relief rather than directly addressing unhelpful beliefs. At this stage of treatment a short-term strategy – known as distraction – may be employed.

The rationale for the use of distraction is to overcome the effects of rumination which interfere with the client's ability to make use of therapy: to provide some distance from frequent upsetting thoughts affecting concentration and attention; and to enable the client to discover their ability to influence and lift their mood (Fennell 1989). A directive approach may be necessary as a temporary measure (Fennell *et al.* 1987). The meaning which the client attaches to the effects of distraction should be checked to guard against 'cognitive avoidance' (Fennell 1989, Gelder 1997). Distraction should be dropped as soon as it has achieved its purpose as in the following example.

Between her first and second appointment Mira's mood deteriorated. She found it difficult to focus her attention on the session as she was preoccupied with thoughts such as 'I can't cope, I'll never be any better. I am a failure'. Mira was encouraged to try a behavioural experiment using distraction techniques to see if it would be possible to produce a slight shift in mood and to act against the belief that she was 'completely unable' to have any impact on controlling fluctuations in her mood.

Mira rated her mood at the start of the experiment as 1/10. She was invited to describe a picture on the wall in as much detail as she could for several minutes. Initially prompts such as were given to sustain her attention. At the end of the experiment Mira noticed that her mood had risen to

3/10 enabling her to focus on the session. She noticed a glimmer of hope that she could have some control over her mood. Further experiments were carried out to test this belief but distraction was only used in session on this occasion. A scale of 0–100% may be used to help the client monitor subtle fluctuations in mood even more effectively.

Activity scheduling

In CBT, diaries are used to monitor how the client spends their time on an hour-by-hour basis. This form of self-monitoring provides useful data on overall levels of activity and demonstrates links between current activity levels and mood. When Mira recognised these links she started to see that adjustments in her activity levels could give her more control over her mood (Fennell 1989). Each activity was rated out of 10 for pleasure (P) and mastery (M). Adjustments were made to increase meaningful and pleasurable activities, which lead to an increase in energy levels and a sense of achievement.

Mira's initial goal was to increase her energy so that she could enjoy being with her children. A graded task assignment based on her hierarchy of preferred occupations was used to build an increased sense of self-efficacy and hope. Recent studies on behavioural activation suggest detailed assessment of individual maintaining factors present in the client's environment is required. This is intended to create opportunities to reinforce non-depressive behaviours (Martell *et al.* 2001, Hopko *et al.* 2003). This seems to link closely with an occupational therapist's attention to analysing facilitating and inhibiting factors operating in the client's social and occupational environment (Kielhofner 2002).

In occupational therapy, feedback loops resulting from engagement with a task, such as playing games in the park with the children, are thought to have the capacity to change the client's cognition and information processing styles. The experience of involvement in occupation is seen as a naturalistic learning tool, which binds together cognition, emotion and action (Kolb 1984, Garrison 2002). The formulation assists in understanding and mapping the dynamic nature of these factors.

When Mira had developed sufficient confidence in using tools to reduce symptoms, the focus of therapy shifted to examine her cognitions more closely. Padesky (1993) states that the timing and sequence of introducing change strategies is crucial in CBT. Repeated thought records were used to capture key negative automatic thoughts and assumptions (Greenberger and Padesky 1995). Collaborative discussion on testing out thoughts and beliefs will prepare the client to adopt a curious, objective, scientific approach to establishing and testing their use and validity (Bennett-Levy 2003).

Guided discovery is a style of questioning used as a tool to assist the client in identifying unhelpful thinking styles and behaviours. These are jointly evaluated to determine their role in maintaining difficulties (see Padesky and Greenberger 1995, p.10 for examples of guided discovery). To assess and understand the impact of cognitive factors on occupational performance it is important to identify indi-vidual differences in appraisals. Appraisals are influenced by the interplay between the person's moods, his or her view of the *context* of the event or task, and past experience. Specific interpretations will lead to particular emotions. The principle of specificity (Salkovskis 1996) is illustrated by the following example.

Mira described experiencing a shift in mood as she worked on sending an email. The computer locked up. Her automatic thoughts in this situation were 'It's all my fault; this shows that I will never be able to manage even simple tasks. I might as well give up. There is no way I am going to try this again. I am getting worse.'

Then Mira noticed that her attention was focused on perceived loss of skills leading to low mood, helplessness and eventual disengagement from the task. She also experienced physical changes including increased lethargy, which interfered with the flow of her performance. She saw this as further evidence that she was 'incapable'. Mira continued to churn these thoughts over, feeling even more depressed.

Mira compared this with her husband's recent appraisal of his computer locking up at work. He described thinking, 'What the hell is going on, they must have altered the settings again'. He felt frustrated with a slight sense of injustice and indignant anger. He then had an energetic conversation with the computer staff and was given advice, which he put into action. The shift in his mood lasted for about 15 minutes. Mira noticed the effect of specific thoughts which made her more depressed, interfered with her problem-solving ability and attention to the task which then strengthened her belief that she was 'incapable.' Understanding the role played by these thoughts led to examining strategies she could use to interrupt, step back and evaluate these thoughts rather than accepting them as completely true. See Bennett-Levy (2003) for discussion on the use of thought records and behavioural experiments at this stage.

Homework setting

One of the characteristics of CBT is the emphasis placed on assignments set between sessions. The rationale for homework is:

- it promotes the autonomy of the client;
- it prepares the person to become his or her own therapist;
- it provides new information to be tested;
- there is continuation of the therapy between sessions.

Burns and Spangler (2000) suggest that homework setting and compliance with homework tasks produce a significant reduction in symptoms of depression during treatment. Engagement in homework assignments between sessions is seen as a strategy which is likely to boost therapeutic effect. Although the content of homework was not identified in this study, the aims of homework setting in

CBT are to gather information through conducting surveys, reflecting and feed-back on self-help material, or engaging in behavioural experiments, to analyse and evaluate existing beliefs and assumptions.

Managing setbacks

Mira returned to work part-time and found that some of her original problems were reactivated. Homework was agreed following exploration of a thought record, where Mira's specific prediction 'I can't tell my manager that I have too much work' led to a lowered mood rated as 80% depressed. Mira tested out the prediction that she would be rejected if she set any limits on the demands made on her. She rated the strength of this belief as 90%. At the next session she noted that her predictions had not been evident and work colleagues appeared to treat her with greater respect. This led to a shift from 80% to 30% intensity in low mood.

The implication for occupational therapists is that setting homework in an overt and detailed manner is likely to lead to increased symptom reduction. Strategies and skills are tested out to see how effective they are over a range of circumstances in the client's life. Feedback and joint discussion help refine how strategies are used. For Mira, the skill of assertion was a key factor leading to an increased sense of efficacy and control in her work role. The CTS-R (Blackburn *et al.* 2001) provides questions to check understanding of the meaning and purpose of homework assignments.

Problem-solving

Occupational therapists use a range of problem-solving strategies to identify, resolve difficulties and restore function (Hagedorn 1997). Problem-solving is an integral and fundamental part of the occupational therapy process and involves a self-help aspect (Fisher 2003). Studies which explore the evidence for the use of problem-solving are therefore of particular interest here. Mynors-Wallis *et al.* (2000) concluded from a randomised controlled trial of antidepressant medication treatment for major depression in primary care versus problem-solving treatment versus a combination of these therapies, that both treatments reduced depressive symptoms. A combination of the therapies did not provide an enhanced result.

Although the mechanism through which problem-solving yields results remains unclear, a hypothesis was made that problem-solving may work through motivating clients to re-engage in activities (Mynors-Wallis 2002). Unless the problem-solving process translates into action to overcome difficulties in every-day life, there is unlikely to be any impact. This is a potential area of research for occupational therapists. It is important to explore the problem-solving style used by the client while depressed. The client's problem-solving may be limited by an increased emphasis on avoiding the possibility of further loss in the future (Leahy

2003). A more detailed critique of problem-solving elements is provided by Roth and Fonaghy (2005, p. 126).

Outcome of therapy

Outcome studies conducted by Beck *et al.* (1979) provide evidence that cognitive therapy reduces relapse and the risk of recurrence of depressive symptoms. Follow-up studies demonstrate that out-patients receiving cognitive therapy for treatment of major depressive episodes relapse less frequently than patients treated with anti-depressant medication, which had been discontinued (Blackburn *et al.* 1986, Simons *et al.* 1986, Evans *et al.* 1992, Shea *et al.* 1992). The provision of cognitive therapy following symptom reduction resulting from medication reduces relapse and recurrence (Fava *et al.* 1996, Fava *et al.* 1998). A combination of ongoing treatment with anti-depressant medication and the addition of cognitive therapy, after a partial response to medication, produced a marked reduction in the rates of relapse (Paykel *et al.* 1999). A Cochrane review states that cognitive therapy combined with anti-depressants reduced relapse rates for people with residual depression as measured at one-year follow-up. Longer-term follow-up studies are needed to ensure gains are maintained (Churchill *et al.* 2000).

These points show that occupational therapists need to pay particular attention to working collaboratively on identifying any remaining vulnerability factors and devising a plan to help the client act against factors such as a tendency to believe all criticism rather than evaluate it.

Prevention of relapse

This aspect of treatment is essential as the rate of recurrence in depression is fairly high (Sainsbury Centre for Mental Health 2005). A current hypothesis suggests that modifying unhelpful aspects of cognitions will reduce vulnerability to relapse in the future (Scott 1996). Further research is required to identify the specific processes of CBT which impact on relapse (Teasdale *et al.* 2001). Greater attention is being paid to analysing the effects of mindfulness mediation which help the person to 'decentre' from ruminative styles of thinking (Teasdale *et al.* 2000).

Key skills in relapse prevention

- To assist clients in creating their own personalised relapse prevention plan.
- To identify individual early warning signs and a step-by-step plan for dealing with each.
- To provide the most up-to-date formulation detailing potential depressive cues and triggers with the person's usual style of responding to these cues.

   To reformulate, highlighting alternative responses, which the client has tested out and found effective.
   To share the plan with carers if the client feels this is helpful.
   To devise an action plan for managing setbacks.
   To build helpful strategies into the client's everyday routine.

To assist in prevention of relapse, reminders of self-help information, which Mira had found helpful were included 'overcoming depression' (Gilbert 1997); and sleep hygiene information (www.livinglifetothefull.com 2005).

The first page of the relapse prevention plan should include a summary of key skills and resources which the client has tested and found of use in managing setbacks. This should be arranged and graded in a logical order so that the person can easily select the most relevant option on occasions when concentration may be lowered. At the end of her therapy Mira commented that the most important skill she had gained was the ability to step back from unhelpful thoughts and dismiss their power to create feelings of dread in her. This skill is likely to act against the fear of low mood occurring in the future. At the end of therapy the relapse prevention plan acts as a reminder to help the client continue to see thoughts as mental events to be tested for accuracy rather than as 'aspects of self or direct reflections of truth' (Teasdale *et al.* 2002).

Follow up appointments are essential to check how far the client's confidence has developed in applying the strategies learned during therapy without further need for a therapist and to fine tune the relapse prevention plan further.

Discussion

Occupational therapists need to continue to analyse empirical evidence for treatment strategies used in CBT for depression. Duncan (2006) suggests that the cognitive-behavioural model is compatible with, and can enhance existing models used by occupational therapists. Strategies used may therefore be seen as 'legitimate therapeutic tools' (Mosey 1996). Selection of the cognitive-behavioural model will be determined according to how far the client sees this as an acceptable form of intervention to address problems and improve quality of life (Mayers 2000). The NICE guidelines (2004) promote the use of CBT as part of the stepped care model for treating depression. Training in CBT is needed to ensure that treatment protocols are adhered to; and to gauge adaptations which would individualise therapy. This is required to apply CBT at every applicable level of the stepped care process (Davison 2000).

Occupational therapists need to continue to question the evidence base to develop reflexive practice selecting effective and acceptable forms of treatment and offering choices which are most relevant to suit individual needs. The therapeutic relationship is of crucial value and must not be overlooked, particularly in overcoming any feelings of shame and stigma which may act against engagement in therapy.

Recommendations

Occupational therapists wishing to apply CBT techniques as a course of treatment for depression need to pursue training and access supervision. Further details may be gained from the British Association of Behavioural and Cognitive Psychotherapists (BABCP) website (www.babcp.com).

References

American Psychiatric Association (2000) *Diagnostic and Statistical Manual of Mental Disorders* (4th edn., text revision) Washington DC: American Psychiatric Association.

Bandura, A. (1997) *Self-Efficacy: The Exercise of Control*. New York: Cambridge University Press.

Beck, A.T. (1967) *Depression: Causes and Treatment*. Philadelphia, PA: University of Pennsylvania Press.

Beck, A.T. (1976) *Cognitive Therapy and the Emotional Disorders*. New York: International Universities Press.

Beck, A.T., Ward, C.H., Mendelson, M., Mock, J. and Erbaugh, J. (1961) An inventory for measuring depression. *Archives of General Psychiatry*. **4**: 561–71.

Beck, A.T., Rush, A.J., Shaw, B.F. and Emery, G. (1979) *Cognitive Therapy of Depression*. New York: The Guilford Press.

Bennett-Levy, J. (2003) Mechanisms of change in cognitive therapy: The case of automatic thought records and behavioural experiments. *Behavioural and Cognitive Psychotherapy*. **31**: 261–77.

Betancourt, J., Green, A. and Carrillo, J. (2002) *Cultural Competence in Health Care: Emerging Frameworks and Practical Approaches*. Field Report, Commonwealth Fund. Available at: www.cmwf.org (accessed 23/11/05).

Blackburn, I.M., Eunson, K.M. and Bishop, S. (1986) A two year naturalistic follow up of depressed patients treated with cognitive therapy, pharmacotherapy, and a combination of both. *Journal of Affective Disorders*. **10**: 67–75.

Blackburn, I.M., James, I., Milne, D., Baker, C., Standart, S., Garland, A. and Reichelt, K. (2001) The Revised Cognitive Therapy Scale (CTS-R): psychometric properties. *Behavioural and Cognitive Psychotherapy*. **29**: 431–46.

Blenkiron, P. (1999) Who is suitable for cognitive behavioural therapy? *Journal of the Royal Society of Medicine*. **92**: 222–9.

Burns, D.D. and Spangler, D. (2000) Does psychotherapy homework lead to improvements in depression in cognitive-behavioral therapy or does improvement lead to increased homework compliance? *Journal of Consulting and Clinical Psychology*. **68**: 46–56.

Butler, G. (1999) Clinical formulation. In: Bellack, A.S. and Herson, M. (eds) *Comprehensive Clinical Psychology*. Oxford: Pergamon Press, **6**: 1–24.

Churchill, R., Wessely, S. and Lewis, G. (2000) Pharmacotherapy and psychotherapy for depression. Protocol for Cochrane Review. In: *The Cochrane Library*, Issue 4. Oxford: Update Software.

Davison, G. (2000) Stepped care doing more with less? *Journal of Consulting and Clinical Psychology*, **68**: 580–5.

Doris, K., Ebmeier, K. and Shajahan, P. (1999) Depressive illness. *The Lancet*. **354**: 1369–82.

Duncan, E.A.S. (2006) The cognitive-behavioural frame of reference. In: Duncan, E.A.S. (ed.) *Foundations for Practice in Occupational Therapy* (4th edn.) Oxford: Elsevier Churchill Livingstone, pp. 217–32.

Evans, D., Hollon, S.D., DeRubeis, R.J., Piasecki, J.M., Grove, W.M., Garvey, M.J. and Tuason, V.B. (1992) Differential relapse following cognitive therapy and pharmacotherapy for depression. *Archives of General Psychiatry*. **49**: 802–8.

Fava, G., Grandi S., Zielezny, M., Rafanelli, C. and Canestrari, R. (1996) Four year outcome for cognitive behavioral treatment of residual symptoms in major depression. *American Journal of Psychiatry*. **153**: 945–7.

Fava, G., Rafanelli, C., Grandi, S., Conti, S. and Belluardo, P. (1998) Prevention of recurrent depression with cognitive behavioral therapy: preliminary findings. *Archives of General Psychiatry*. **55**: 816–20.

Fennell, M. (1989) Depression. In: Hawton, K., Salkovskis, P., Kirk, J. and Clark, D. (eds) *Cognitive Behaviour Therapy for Psychiatric Problems: A Practical Guide*. Oxford: Oxford University Press.

Fennell, M.J.V. (1997) Working with low self-esteem: a cognitive perspective. *Behavioural and Cognitive Psychotherapy*. **25**: 1–25.

Fennell, M.J., Teasdale, J.D., Jones, S. and Damle, A. (1987) Distraction in neurotic and endogenous depression: an investigation of negative thinking in major depressive disorder. *Psychological Medicine*. **17**: 441–52.

Fisher, A.G. (2003) *Assessment of Motor and Process Skills, Vol 2, User Manual* (5th edn.). Fort Collins: Three Star Press.

Garrison, J.W. (2002) Habits as social tools in context. *The Occupational Journal of Research*. Supplement. **2**: 115–75.

Gelder, M. (1997) The Scientific foundations of cognitive behaviour therapy. In. Clark, D.M. and Fairburn, C.G. (eds) *Science and Practice of Cognitive Behaviour Therapy*. Oxford: Oxford University Press.

Gilbert, P. (1997) *Overcoming Depression: a Self-help Guide Using Cognitive Behavioural Techniques*. London: Robinson.

Gilbert, P. (2000) Social Mentalities: Internal 'social' conflict and the role of inner warmth and compassion in cognitive therapy. In: Gilbert, P. and Bailey, K.G. *Genes on the Couch: Explorations in Evolutionary Psychotherapy*. Philadelphia: Brunner Routledge.

Gilbert, P., Gilbert, J. and Sanghera, J. (2004) A focus group exploration of the impact of izzat, shame, subordination entrapment on mental health and service use in South Asian women living in Derby. *Mental Health, Religion and Culture*. **7**: 109–30.

Gilbody, S.M., House, A.O. and Sheldon, T.A. (2001) Routinely administered questionnaires for depression and anxiety: systematic review. *BMJ*. **322**: 406–9.

Greenberger, D. and Padesky, C.A. (1995) *Mind Over Mood: Change How You Feel by Changing the Way You Think*. New York: The Guilford Press.

Gutman, S.A. and Hayes, J.L. (2002) Unipolar depression: A literature review of the most current epidemiological theories. *Occupational Therapy in Mental Health*. **18**: 45–77.

Hagedorn, R. (1997) *Foundations for Practice In Occupational Therapy*. New York: Churchill Livingstone.

Hopko, D., Lejuez, C.W., Ruggiero, K.J. and Eifert, G.H. (2003) Contemporary behavioural activation treatments for depression: Procedures, principles and progress. *Clinical Psychology Review.* **23**: 699–717.

Kielhofner, G. (2002) *A Model of Human Occupation: Theory and Application* (3rd edn.). Baltimore: Lippincott Williams & Wilkins.

Kielhofner, G., Mallinson, T., Crawford, C., Nowak, M., Rigby, M., Hening, A., and Walens, D. (1998). *A User's Manual for the Occupational Performance History Interview. (Version 2.0) OPHI-II.* Chicago: The Model of Human Occupation Clearinghouse, Department of Occupational Therapy,University of Illinois at Chicago.

Kolb, D.A. (1984) *Experiential Learning: Experience as the Source of Learning and Development.* Englewood Cliffs, NJ: Prentice Hall.

Kusznir, A. and Scott, E. (1999) The challenges of client-centred practice in mental health settings. In: Sumsion, T. (ed.) *Client-centred Practice in Occupational Therapy: A Guide to Implementation.* New York: Churchill Livingstone.

Layard Lord, R. (2004) Mental health: Britain's biggest social problem? Available at: www.strategy.gov.uk/downloads/files/mh_layard.pdf (accessed 13/12/05)

Leahy, R.L. (ed.) (2003) *Overcoming Roadblocks in Cognitive-Behavioral Therapy.* New York: Guilford.

Living life to the full . . . helping you to help yourself (2005). www.livinglifetothefull.com (accessed 5/10/05).

Martell, C.R., Addis, M.E. and Jacobson, N.S. (2001) *Depression in Context: Strategies for Guided Action.* New York: WW Norton.

Mattingly, C. (1994) *Clinical Reasoning: Forms of Enquiry in a Therapeutic Practice.* Philadelphia: F.A. Davis.

Mayers, C.A. (2000) Quality of life: priorities for people with enduring mental health problems. *British Journal of Occupational Therapy.* **63**: 591–7.

Mee, J., Sumsion, T. and Craik, C. (2004) Mental health clients confirm the value of occupation in building competence and self-identify. *British Journal of Occupational Therapy* **67**: 225–33.

Moore, R.G. and Garland, A. (2003) *Cognitive Therapy for Chronic and Persistent Depression.* Chichester: Wiley.

Moorey, S. (1996) When bad things happen to rational people: cognitive therapy in adverse life circumstances. In: Salkovskis, P.M. (ed.) *Frontiers of Cognitive Therapy.* New York: Guilford, pp. 266–79.

Morgan, S. (2000) *Clinical Risk Management: a clinical tool and practitioner manual.* London: Sainsbury Centre for Mental Health.

Mosey, A.C. (1996) *Psychosocial Components of Occupational Therapy.* Philadelphia: Lippincott Williams and Wilkins.

Mynors-Wallis, L. (2002) Does problem-solving treatment work through resolving problems? *Psychological Medicine.* **32**: 1315–19.

Mynors-Wallis, L., Gath, D., Day, A. and Baker, F. (2000) Randomised controlled trial of problem solving treatment, antidepressant medication and combined treatment for major depression in primary care. *BMJ* **320**: 26–30.

National Institute for Clinical Excellence (2004) *Depression: Management of depression in primary and secondary care. Clinical Guideline 23.* London: NICE.

Padesky, C.A. (1993) Schema as self-prejudice. *International Cognitive Therapy Newsletter.* 5/**6**: 16–17.

Padesky, C.A. and Greenberger, D. (1995) *Clinician's Guide to Mind Over Mood.* New York: The Guilford Press.

Papadopoulos, I. (2006) *Transcultural Health and Social Care: Developing Culturally Competent Practitioners.* Edinburgh: Churchill Livingstone.

Paykel, E.S., Scott, J., Teasdale, J.D., Johnson, A.L., Garland, A., Moore, R., Jenaway, A., Cornwall, P.L., Hayhurst, H., Abbott, R. and Pope, M. (1999) Prevention of relapse in residual depression by cognitive therapy: a controlled trial. *Archives of General Psychiatry.* **56**: 829–35.

Paykel, E.S. (2002) Achieving gains beyond response. *Acta Psychiatric Scandinavia Supplement.* 106 (Suppl. 415): 12–17.

Persons, J.B. (1989) *Cognitive Therapy in Practice*: *A Case Formulation Approach.* New York: W.W. Norton & Co.

Richards, D. and McDonald, B. (1990) *Behavioural Psychotherapy: a Handbook for Nurses.* Oxford, Heinemann.

Roth, A. and Fonaghy, P. (2005) *What works for whom? A critical review of psychotherapy research* (2nd edn.). New York: The Guilford Press.

Safran, J.D., Segal, Z.V., Shaw, B.F. and Vallis, T.M. (1996) Patient selection for short term cognitive therapy. In: J.D. Safran and Segal, Z.V. *Interpersonal Process in Cognitive Therapy.* New York: Basic Books, pp. 226–38.

Sainsbury Centre for Mental Health (2005) *The Neglected Majority: Developing Intermediate Mental Health Care in Primary Care.* London: SCMH.

Salkovskis, P.M. (1996) Avoidance behaviour is motivated by threat beliefs: A possible resolution of the cognition-behaviour debate. In: Salkovskis, P.M. (ed.) *Trends in Cognitive and Behavioural Therapies.* New York: John Wiley and Sons.

Sashidharan, S.P. (2003) *Inside, Outside, Improving Mental Health Services for Black and Ethnic Minority Communities in England.* London: National Institute for Mental Health in England. Available at: www.dh.gov.uk/Home/fs/en (accessed on 23/06/05).

Scott, J. (1996) Cognitive therapy of affective disorders: a review. *Journal of Affective Disorders.* **37**: 1–11.

Scott, J., Cole, A. and Eccleston, D. (1991) Dealing with persistent abnormalities of mood. *International Review of Psychiatry.* **3**: 19–33.

Shea, M.T., Elkin, I., Imber, S.D., Sotsky, F.M., Watkins, J.T., Collins, J.F., Pilkonis, P.A., Beckham, E., Glass, R., Dolan, R.T. and Parloff, M.B. (1992) Course of depressive symptoms over follow up: findings from the NIMH treatment of depression collaborative research program. *Archives of General Psychiatry.* **49**: 782–7.

Simons, A.D., Murphy, G.E., Levine, J.L. and Wetzal, R.D. (1986) Cognitive therapy and pharmacotherapy for depression: sustained improvement over one year. *Archives of General Psychiatry.* **43**: 43–50.

Snyder, C.R. (2000) *Handbook of Hope.* San Diego: Academic Press.

Tarrier, N. and Calam, R. (2002) New developments in cognitive-behavioural case formulation, epidemiological, systemic and social context: an integrative approach. *Behavioural and Cognitive Psychotherapy.* **30**: 311–28.

Teasdale, J.D., Williams, J.M.G., Soulsby, J.M., Segal, Z.V., Ridgeway, V.A. and Lau, M.A. (2000) Prevention of relapse/recurrence in major depression by mindfulness-based cognitive therapy. *Journal of Consulting and Clinical Psychology.* **68**: 615–23.

Teasdale, J.D., Moore, R.G., Hayhurst, H., Scott, J., Pope, M. and Paykel, E.S. (2001) How does cognitive therapy prevent relapse in residual depression? evidence from a controlled trial. *Journal of Consulting and Clinical Psychology.* **69**: 347–57.

Teasdale, J.D., Pope, M., Moore, R.G., Hayhurst, H., Williams, S. and Segal, Z.V. (2002) Metacognitive awareness and prevention of relapse in depression: empirical evidence. *Journal of Consulting and Clinical Psychology.* **70**: 275–87.

Vallis, T.M, Howes, J.L. and Standage, K. (2000) Is cognitive therapy suitable for treating individuals with personality dysfunction? *Cognitive Therapy and Research.* **24**: 595–606.

Waddington, L. (2002) The therapy relationship in cognitive therapy: a review. *Behavioural and Cognitive Psychotherapy.* **30**: 179–92.

Westen, D. and Morrison, K. (2001) A multidimensional meta-analysis of treatments for depression, panic, and generalized anxiety disorder: an empirical examination of the status of empirically supported therapies. *Journal of Consulting and Clinical Psychology.* **69**: 875–99.

Whitney, D.K., Kusznir, A. and Dixie, A. (2002) Women with depression: the importance of social, psychological and occupational factors in illness and recovery. *Journal of Occupational Science.* **9**: 20–7.

Williams, C. and Garland, A. (2002) A cognitive-behavioural therapy assessment model for use in everyday clinical practice. *Advances in Psychiatric Treatment.* **8**: 172–9.

World Health Organization (1992) *The Tenth Revision of the International Classification of Diseases and Related Health Problems.* Geneva: WHO.

Yerxa, E.J. (2000) Confessions of an occupational therapist who became a detective. *British Journal of Occupational Therapy.* **63**: 192–9.

Zuroff, D.C., Sotsky, S.M., Martin, D.J., Sanislow III, C.A., Blatt, S.J., Krupnick, J.L. and Simmens, S. (2000) Relation of therapeutic alliance and perfectionism to outcome in brief outpatient treatment of depression. *Journal of Consulting and Clinical Psychology.* **68**: 114–24.

4: Occupational therapy interventions for someone experiencing severe and enduring mental illness

Lindsay Rigby and Ian Wilson

Health professionals are increasingly guided by research to determine the effectiveness of their clinical practice (Murphy *et al.* 1998, Popay and Williams 1998, Glasziou *et al.* 2001, Khan *et al.* 2003). Occupational therapists, as professionals who are integral to the effectiveness of multi-disciplinary teams, must have an awareness of the application of evidence-based assessments and interventions (CRD 2001). There is an expanding body of research in psychosocial interventions (PSI) to support the implementation of innovative, holistic and collaborative approaches to help people with psychosis and their families (Baguley and Baguley 1999).

For clients with psychotic symptoms, medication has been the first line of treatment offered since the advent of neuroleptics 50 years ago. Despite the benefits gained from medication, it has limitations. Non-compliance has been attributed as the reason for a 30–50% increase in hospital admissions (Kane 1985). In a study by Finn *et al.* (1990) with clients who were agreeable to take medication, the side-effects were felt to be as distressing as the symptoms for which they were being prescribed. There is also a proportion of clients for whom medication has little benefit (Brown and Herz 1989), or who continue to experience residual positive psychotic symptoms (Curson *et al.* 1988). Johnstone *et al.* (1984) found that after a period of 5–9 years on medication, 50% of clients continued to experience psychotic symptoms. It therefore seems appropriate to consider other treatments that might be offered in conjunction with medication regimens. The National Institute of Clinical Excellence (NICE) has used evidence from randomised controlled trials and systematic reviews of the literature to establish guidelines for the treatment of schizophrenia, which recommend the incorporation of psychosocial interventions that include both family interventions, and cognitive behavioural therapy in the treatment offered to patients and carers (NICE 2002).

PSI have become a familiar concept in most mental health settings and refer to those collaborative interventions that have an impact on the psychological and social experiences of clients and carers. Such interventions involve engagement with clients and their carers, the process of completing a comprehensive assessment, case management, cognitive-behavioural therapy, early interventions and relapse prevention in psychosis and family interventions (Baguley and Baguley 1999). The aim of such interventions is to manage symptoms and experiences associated with severe and enduring illness using an evidence-based approach. For individuals with residual symptoms of psychosis, Beck (1952) had successfully utilised psychological therapy to reduce distress caused by delusional beliefs. Clinicians and researchers have investigated interventions to reduce symptoms and prevent or delay relapse, first through single-case studies utilising behavioural techniques (e.g. Lindsley 1959, Nydegger 1972) and by use of cognitive techniques (Watts *et al.* 1973, Milton *et al.* 1978, Chadwick and Lowe 1990). Randomised controlled trials (e.g. Kuipers *et al.* 1997, Tarrier *et al.* 1998, Sensky *et al.* 2000) have tested the efficacy of such approaches under tightly controlled conditions. Family interventions have been systematically reviewed in the Cochrane database (Pharoah *et al.* 2006), as have cognitive-behavioural interventions for individuals (Cormac *et al.* 2006). The evidence base for PSI continues to develop as researchers are becoming increasingly aware interventions that have been found to be effective must now be applied to clinical practice.

Occupational therapists are able to utilise the core skills of systematic and comprehensive assessments to develop specific and collaborative goals that are essential to the delivery of psychosocial interventions. Clearly, the core skills of occupational therapy reflect the basis of psychosocial interventions as they both facilitate and develop the individual's strengths and abilities to maintain independent living skills and to cope with experiences associated with severe mental illness. Many postgraduate occupational therapists have undergone further training in psychosocial interventions to build on these existing core skills.

Training in psychosocial interventions has become increasingly accessible over the last few years for mental health professionals who have a recognised qualification in nursing, occupational therapy or social work. In the Northwest of England, the COPE Initiative recruited and trained over 300 mental health professionals over three years (Bradshaw *et al.* 2002) and continues to provide high-quality training in PSI. Newly qualified professionals are not expected to have a detailed knowledge of PSI (see Table 4.1). However, there is a clear trend towards the incorporation of psychosocial concepts in the undergraduate training curriculum. Many mental health trusts are also providing local training initiatives at certificate and diploma levels as part of in-house service training programmes.

Task box 1

- Find the NICE guidelines (www.nice.org.uk).
- Develop a search by using the keyword schizophrenia. Then click the icon which allows you to open the PDF of the full copy of the published document.
- List all the psychosocial interventions for schizophrenia recommended in the guidelines.

Table 4.1 Psychosocial interventions and the evidence base.

Components of Psychosocial Interventions		
Intervention	**Evidence Base**	**Systematic review**
Global and specific assessment of mental state	Gamble and Brennon (2006) Ryrie (2000)	
Assessment of activities of daily living/social functioning/quality of life	Oliver et al. (1997), Law et al. (1990), Birchwood et al. (1990)	
CBT for psychosis	Tarrier et al. (1998), Kuipers et al. (1997), Tarrier et al. (2004), Sensky et al. (2000)	Cormac et al. (2006), Pilling et al. (2002).
Family interventions	Leff et al. (1982, 1985), Falloon (1985), Hogarty et al. (1986), Kuipers and Bebbington (1985)	Mari and Streiner (1994), Pilling et al. (2002), Pharoah et al. (2006)
Early intervention	Morrison et al. (2004), Johannessen (2001)	
Coping strategy enhancement	Tarrier et al. (1993, 1998)	
Relapse prevention	Falloon et al. (1993), Birchwood et al. (1998), Birchwood and MacMillan (1993), Herz et al. (2000)	
Medication management and motivational interviewing	Kemp et al. (1996), Rollnick and Miller (1995), Pekkala and Merinder (2006)	
Case management	Rossler et al. (1995)	Marshall et al. (2006)
Development of social and employment skills	Lehman et al. (1998), Marwaha and Johnson (2005)	Robertson et al. (2006), Crowther et al. (2003), Rebeiro (1998)

The occupational therapy pathway

The incorporation of psychosocial interventions into occupational therapy practice presents the opportunity for the profession to integrate existing evidence-based practice into the occupational therapy process. This chapter illustrates the delivery of these interventions in a specialist mental health setting – a multi-disciplinary home treatment team in a diverse inner-city environment. We have developed a case study that guides the reader through the occupational therapy process while focusing specifically upon evidence-based interventions incorporated into assessments and interventions implemented with both the client and his carers. The occupational therapy team has developed a pathway to identify needs based on the Canadian Model of Occupational Performance (CMOP, Law *et al.* 1991). This client-centred model presents the person as an integrated spiritual whole incorporating mental, physical and socio-cultural aspects of performance, while also considering environmental factors that might affect the ability of the individual to perform to their perceived potential in the functional areas of self-care, productivity and leisure (Law *et al.* 1990, 1991).

Example of practice

Background

Bob is in his early 20s and is currently living with his mother and father. Bob first developed psychotic symptoms when he was 18 years old, while he was studying for exams. However, he only came to the attention of services several months later when his symptoms deteriorated and his family could no longer cope with his distress and unpredictable behaviour. His family eventually contacted their general practitioner (GP) for an urgent appointment. A referral was made to a psychiatrist, who assessed him as an out-patient and immediately contacted the home treatment team to organise an admission to this service.

Home treatment teams were established as a result of a government initiative to provide an alternative to in-patient admission for people who experience acute episodes of mental illness. The multi-disciplinary home treatment team is available 24 hours a day, seven days a week for clients suffering from either a relapse of a enduring illness or presenting with a first episode of a psychotic illness and who are perceived as being at risk. The initial focus of intervention is engagement of clients followed by assessment, symptom reduction, support to clients and carers and relapse prevention within the framework of the Care Programme Approach (Department of Health (DoH) 1990).

Referral, engagement and assessment

A benefit of research is the development of standardised baseline assessment scales (e.g. Overall and Gorham 1962, Krawiecka *et al.* 1977, Andreasen 1984, Chadwick *et al.* 2000), enabling the measurement of treatment (Chadwick and Lowe 1990). Early case studies in psychosocial research were small and had many methodological weaknesses. More recent studies have included the use of standardised assessments, randomisation of clients, the use of control groups, the use of 'blind' raters and the incorporation of follow-up assessments to evaluate the efficacy of interventions. There have recently been moves to translate efficacious interventions from research trials into effective mainstream clinical practice. The process of assessment enables clinicians to gain a detailed understanding of the components of a psychological reaction and to consider the most appropriate treatment intervention.

On admission to the home treatment team Bob and the allocated occupational therapist collaboratively identified and prioritised specific functional and occupational needs using an occupational therapy referral form based on the CMOP (Law *et al.* 1991). From a list of problems, two specific problem areas were prioritised using the standardised and validated Canadian Model of Occupational Performance Measure (COPM, Law *et al.* 1994) and translated into needs using a goal-setting approach (Park 2003, Goal setting in occupational therapy: evaluating client-centred outcomes [course handout] London: Harrison Associates). The first of these was a need for Bob to find ways of coping with distressing malevolent auditory hallucinations that were derogatory and commanding and prevented him from going to the sports centre, an activity he had previously enjoyed.

Second, Bob said that arguments took place at home concerning his difficulty in getting out of bed and attending to his appearance. He acknowledged that he had neglected his personal care and was keen to make more 'effort' to improve his appearance. He believed that if he did, the friction in the family would improve and he might feel more confident about resuming some of his previous activities. Bob was dissatisfied with his current ability to cope with the voices he was experiencing and his self-care, both of which he rated as 'low' on the COPM. We devised a written contract with Bob for the implementation of both individual and family work. The contract was collaboratively developed to identify the length, frequency and duration of session and clarified issues of confidentiality.

The development of a contract assists in the balance of power between the client and therapist to ensure that the client's needs are met and that they are aware of the interventions they will receive. The contract specifically defined both short- and long-term goals that were identified during the assessment process and outlined how these were to be achieved. Dates for the evaluation of the goals were also written into the contract. Both parties signed the contract and copies were provided for Bob to keep.

Task box 2

- Why is the COPM a useful assessment tool in this case study?
- What are the advantages of the COPM?
- What are the drawbacks of using a client-centred assessment tool?

Having identified the areas of need by using the COPM, we needed to gain a more detailed understanding of the distress Bob experienced as a result of his voices and how this distress was preventing him from participating in activities that were meaningful to him. Historically, clinicians were deterred from discussing either delusional content or hallucinatory experiences with patients because it was feared that it might reinforce them. There is, however, no evidence to support this hypothesis. On the contrary, without any other psychological input, clients have found that talking about their psychotic experiences can be beneficial (Bentall 1996).

The Belief About Voices Questionnaire (BAVQ, Chadwick and Birchwood 1995, Chadwick *et al.* 2000) and the Psychotic Symptoms Rating Scale (PSYRATS, Haddock *et al.* 1999) was used to establish the phenomenology of the voices for

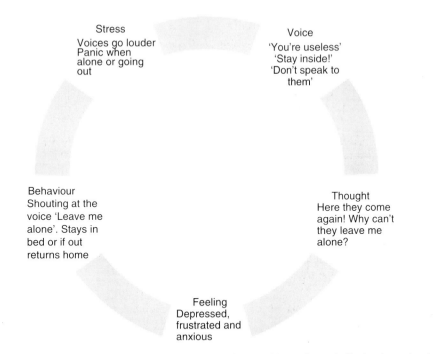

Stress
Voices go louder
Panic when
alone or going
out

Voice
'You're useless'
'Stay inside!'
'Don't speak to
them'

Behaviour
Shouting at the
voice 'Leave me
alone'. Stays in
bed or if out
returns home

Thought
Here they come
again! Why can't
they leave me
alone?

Feeling
Depressed,
frustrated and
anxious

Figure 4.1 Formulation illustrating distress associated with auditory hallucinations developed from the individual assessments.

Bob and to provide a baseline from which to measure the effectiveness of interventions. These are standardised assessments that have been validated with this client group. The Antecedent and Coping Interview (ACI, Tarrier *et al.* 1993 was also completed with Bob. This is a semi-structured interview that elicits emotional reactions, antecedents and consequences of voice hearing experiences. These assessments enabled us to develop an 'understanding' of the problem areas on which to base individual interventions. This 'formulation', a working hypothesis, was collaboratively agreed with Bob and is illustrated in Figure 4.1.

Exploring the evidence of individual interventions

Coping strategy enhancement

Coping is a process whereby an individual examines and evaluates a set of circumstances or experiences as a problem and then attempts to overcome this problem (Table 4.2). It involves the ability to implement personal resources and self-efficacy (Tarrier 2002). The models of stress vulnerability developed by Zubin and Spring (1977) and Nuechterlein and Dawson (1984) acknowledge that those who experience psychotic symptoms are potentially more vulnerable to the impact of stress. The ability to cope positively with such stressful situations is, however, a protective factor that can inhibit the onset of symptoms.

Table 4.2 Coping strategies for psychosis.

Attention disruption	This involves disrupting the psychotic experience from switching attention away from the symptom or triggers that initiate the symptom. This might involve listening to music, humming, singing or the use of imagery (Carr 1888, Nelson 1991).
Social engagement/ disengagement	The client might withdraw for periods of time until arousal levels decrease or actively engage with others as means of reassurance or distraction
Attention narrowing	Filtering of information and focusing attention by suppression of unwanted thoughts or perceptual experiences (Tarrier 2002)
Reframing of psychosis	Normalisation of symptoms has the effect of both reducing stress and stigma. Alternative explanations of the psychotic experiences might be offered such as assisting the client to attribute voices heard as one's own thought rather than externally to alien sources
Self-affirmation	Encouraging the client to use assertiveness, social skills training and positive memory
Belief modification	Cognitive-behavioural therapy techniques: guided discovery, exploration, re-examination and reattribution (Kingdon and Turkington, 1994)
Reducing physiological arousal	Medication, relaxation, controlled breathing exercises (Fowles 1992)
Increasing structured activity	Activity remediation strategies (Wykes *et al.* 2003), activity scheduling, goal setting and problem solving

Many individuals with psychosis find it very difficult to structure their lives with meaningful activity. Complete resolution of all symptoms is not always possible. However, occupational therapists can play a crucial role in helping clients to get on with their lives despite the problems they experience by developing methods of coping. Symptom reduction and removal, although important, may be no more so for the individual than recovering their own self-efficacy and their ability to function at an optimum level. This is what promotes true 'recovery' from a psychotic illness (Deegan 1998) and should be at the core of occupational therapy intervention for this client group.

In 1989 a Dutch psychiatrist called Marius Romme appeared on a television programme in the Netherlands with a patient who experienced hearing voices. A total of 450 people responded to the programme, and 300 stated, in a questionnaire to elicit coping strategies for the voices they experienced, that they were unable to cope effectively with them, although 150 other respondents did feel able to cope with them and manage them. When a comparison was made between the two groups, those unable to cope with voices generally found them to be negative and aggressive while those who could cope found their voices to be positive and friendly (Romme and Escher 1989). From this study it was established that the process of coping has many variations and dimensions, including the attributed meaning of the voice and the degree of interference or rejection of the voice as internal or as external and alien. The real problem is not so much the hearing of voices as the inability to cope with the experience.

A further study by Tarrier (1987) used the Antecedent and Coping Interview (ACI) to elicit subjective accounts of the psychotic experiences of clients, the emotional reaction to these and the use of coping strategies in response to these experiences. Of the individuals studied, 32% were able to identify antecedents to either the onset or exacerbation of their symptoms. These included specific triggers such as television programmes, social situations, social isolation or internal states such as increased anxiety levels. The response to psychotic experiences was also variable: 72% felt distressed, with 12% of these individuals describing their distress as severe. Those 72% of clients in this study found that at least one of the coping strategies implemented was successful in moderating the symptom experienced. It is clear from observational studies that individuals do attempt to control their symptoms independently to reduce the distressing effects. Falloon and Talbot (1991) identified that those clients experiencing auditory hallucinations used behavioural and cognitive strategies and attempts to lower physiological arousal to control the impact of the voices. Similar coping strategies have also been observed in other studies (Carr 1988, Carter et al. 1996, Dittman and Schüttler 1990).

Research into hallucinations tends to refer to auditory hallucinations, especially in the earlier case studies. For instance, Nydegger (1972) attempted to bring auditory hallucinations under operant control by the withdrawal of social contact if the client failed to take personal responsibility for the content of the auditory hallucination. Green and Preston (1981) observed that when clients are experiencing auditory hallucinations they also present with an accompanying micro-movement of the small speech muscles, known as sub-vocalisation. Margo et al. (1981) conducted a study to ascertain the effect of controlling external stimuli to modify and interrupt sub-vocalisation, in order to have an impact on auditory hallucinations. In an experiment with ten clients and nine different types of auditory stimuli compared to a control group, they found that the most beneficial activity for the voice hearer was reading aloud, especially if the subject matter was meaningful and captured the reader's attention. Other studies have included the use of earplugs, based on the theory that hallucinations arise from a disturbance in the inter-hemispheric transmission of information (Green et al. 1994); and passive and active distraction techniques using personal stereos and mental games (Nelson et al. 1991). In a review of distraction techniques, Haddock et al. (1993) felt them to be useful only if the voices were not negative in nature.

'Focusing' involves the encouragement of the client to focus on the physical characteristics, content and meaning of voices in relation to his/her own thoughts and to elicit the beliefs the client has concerning the presence of the voices (Haddock *et al.* 1993). Fowler and Morley (1989) reported success with five clients in a study using a combination of focusing and distraction techniques. Haddock *et al.* (1998) undertook a comparative study of distraction and focusing in a controlled randomised trial of 19 clients with a diagnosis of schizophrenia. Both groups benefited from the psychological treatments in terms of a decrease in distress levels and disruption to life style. However, the 'focusing' group also improved in terms of their self-esteem, evaluated using the Rosenburg Self Esteem Rating Scale (Rosenburg 1965).

The use of naturalistic coping strategies was investigated by Tarrier *et al.* (1993) and was based on facilitating clients to develop a self-management approach to their psychotic experiences. The aim was to maximise existing coping strategies, modify or remove less helpful methods of coping and to introduce new, potentially effective ones. In order to establish the efficacy of 'coping strategy enhancement' (CSE), as it was termed, it was compared with a problem-solving intervention. Results showed that both were superior at reducing positive symptoms of psychosis when compared with a waiting list control. Of the group receiving CSE, 60% showed a 50% improvement in symptoms compared with only 20% of the problem-solving group. At follow-up, however, there was a drop in the improvement in the CSE group from 60% to 42%. The study also showed that CSE was effective in treating anxiety and delusional beliefs but less so in the treatment of auditory hallucinations.

A later study (Tarrier *et al.* 1998) compared a combination of CSE, problem solving and relapse prevention with supportive counselling and routine care and routine care alone. This study, which involved 25 clients, of whom 18 had hallucinatory experiences, found that cognitive therapy was superior to supportive counselling and routine care, which in turn was superior to routine care alone. Significantly more patients receiving the combination of coping strategy enhancement, problem-solving and relapse prevention showed a reduction of 50% or more in psychotic symptoms than did patients in either of the other conditions. It was not possible from this study to determine which of these three interventions was the most efficacious. A follow-up study found that the effectiveness of the cognitive-behavioral therapy approach had been maintained when comparing this to supportive counselling, especially for delusional beliefs and anxiety (Tarrier *et al.* 1999). The evidence for hallucinations and depression was less convincing. Chadwick and Birchwood (1994) provided a useful piece of research in a study that focused on client's beliefs about voices. They found that it appears to be beliefs about voices rather than the actual content of the voices that is linked to the distress caused by the experience. It appears that changes in beliefs about the voices' omnipotence, purpose and identity can reduce levels of distress.

The negative symptoms of schizophrenia include anhedonia, apathy, poor motivation, inattention and a general reduction of functioning at an emotional, cognitive and social level (Andreasen 1984, Hogg 1996). In a study of 25 clients with a diagnosis of schizophrenia, Mueser *et al.* (1997) showed that those who developed a wider range of coping strategies believed that they were more able to cope with negative symptoms.

In order to achieve the goal of reducing levels of distress when Bob hears voices, CSE was implemented over 6 planned sessions. From the ACI it was identified that Bob became increasingly distressed when his parents were critical and shouted at him. He coped with these arguments by isolating himself in his bedroom, away from his family. However, once alone, he was less able to distract himself from the voices and as a result he felt low in mood. In response to this he drank cans of extra strong beer to 'numb himself'. This in turn exacerbated an existing sense of low self-esteem and self-confidence. When he went out, the voices became commanding in nature, instructing him to go home. He tended to obey the voices and return home. This prevented him from going to the sports centre, exacerbating an existing sense of low self-esteem and a reduction in his confidence level. In addition to standardised assessments, Bob was asked to complete a detailed diary of his experiences in order to ascertain further phenomenological aspects of the voices, including frequency, duration and content. A typical entry in this diary is given in Table 4.3.

Task box 3

- What sort of coping strategies do people use when they experience high stress levels?
- Which of these coping strategies can be unhealthy?
- List the coping strategies which can be used by clients to decrease the distress caused by voices, giving examples of how this could be implemented by Bob
- How could the use of coping strategies be evaluated for their effectiveness?

Initially, the coping strategies implemented by Bob were elicited. Bob was asked to rate the effectiveness of each of the coping strategies on a Likert Scale rated from 1–10 using a diary. He also monitored his alcohol use, arguments and periods of isolation in the diary so that he could make comparisons with all the coping strategies he implemented. The link between stress and an increase in symptoms was explored in relation to the stress/vulnerability model (Zubin and Spring 1977). A rationale was given for developing and/or extending current coping strategies or modifying or reducing ineffective strategies. The less successful strategies or the ones that caused disruption to normal functioning were discussed with a view to reducing or modifying them. These included social withdrawal (staying in bed, refusing to speak to family or friends), shouting at the voices and drinking alcohol to excess. The more effective and reliable strategies were then rehearsed and practised in vivo to increase their potential for controlling the symptom and reducing the amount of distress caused by it. The coping strategies that were reinforced are illustrated in Table 4.4.

The importance of practice and rehearsal was emphasised before new strategies were introduced. Bob was encouraged to continue with his diary to list any stressful situations and rate distress levels in relation to the voices. He was then

Table 4.3 An example of a diary entry by Bob.

Date/time/situation	Tuesday morning. At home with mum. We had a big row because I couldn't get up for a shower Tuesday evening. Tried to walk down the road towards gym
Target problem	I heard a man telling me that I was useless and a ******* waste of time! The voice told me to return home
How did you feel?	Angry, anxious, upset, frustrated
What did you think?	Here we go again. It's not fair, I've been taking my tablets yet it's still happening. It gets worse every time I have a row with mum I can't even manage to go down the road – I'm useless!
What did you do?	Morning – stayed in the bedroom and refused to go downstairs to talk to mum about what had happened Evening – Went home
How did you cope?	Voice got worse for the next 30 minutes then gradually went away. Eventually decided to go to the gym but the voices returned so I started to shout at them when I got to the bedroom and had a few beers to calm me down

Table 4.4 List of coping strategies utilized by Bob.

Cognitive strategies	Attention disruption
	  Listening to the local talk radio programme
	  Listening to music, increased social interaction with friends and family if there is no argument
	Reattribution
	  Re-framing his belief about his voices as his own thoughts
	Self-affirmation
	  Thinking about positive things to look forward to in the future and skills recently acquired

Behavioural strategies	Increasing structured activity
	  Going into the garden rather than walking down the street
	  Playing games on a games console

Physiological strategies	Reducing physiological arousal Taking medication; relaxation; breathing exercises
Sensory strategies	Attention narrowing Wearing headphones to 'block out' voices

asked to list which coping strategies were implemented and to re-rate his distress levels.

The effectiveness of each coping strategy was reviewed. Those strategies that were helpful included the following

- Inviting a friend to go with him to the sports centre.
- Reframing his voices as his own thoughts rather than evil voices.
- Deep breathing when walking towards the gym.
- Listening to the local talk radio channel while getting up in the morning.

Bob then practised these until they gradually became part of a daily routine. The formulation was then collaboratively revisited and revised. The final session explored how Bob might establish control when in unpredictable situations so that he might generalise the techniques learnt to different settings and situations.

Cognitive-behavioural family interventions

The second need identified through the COPM was Bob's difficulties in getting up in the morning and managing his personal care. This was discussed with his family who expressed specific concerns about his ability to shower, shave and change his clothes on a regular basis. Bob's parents became distressed by this and resorted to shouting at him in a critical and hostile manner. They then felt guilty about these frequent arguments. His mother attempted to compensate for these outbursts by running baths for him and laying out his clothes. Bob had become increasingly dependent on her and she said that she found this dependence over-whelming. Cognitive-behavioural family therapy was offered by the authors over a period of 10 sessions to implement psycho-education, problem solving and stress management interventions.

Cognitive-behavioural family interventions have been recognised as an effective treatment option for schizophrenia for many years. Basing therapy on the concepts of expressed emotion (EE, Brown *et al.* 1972), Vaughn and Leff (1976) investigated the importance of high levels of expressed emotion (HEE) on the course and outcome of schizophrenia. An important link was made between stressful factors in a person's environment and the number and nature of subsequent psychotic relapse. There has been a long history of research into cognitive-behavioural family interventions to influence the course of psychosis, using tightly controlled experimental conditions (Leff *et al.* 1985, Falloon *et al.* 1982, 1985, Hogarty *et al.* 1986, Tarrier *et al.* 1988, 1989). In summary these and other studies were able to conclude that successful family intervention can lead to at least a fourfold reduction in relapse rates at one year post-intervention, maintained (though reduced in effectiveness) in subsequent follow-up. It has become clear that offering a combination of medication and family intervention leads to unquestionably superior outcomes for patients with schizophrenia than medication or 'routine care' alone (World Schizophrenia Fellowship 1997, Fadden 1998, Lehman

et al. 1998). Although there have been problems associated with translating efficacy of research into effective services (Fadden 1997), successful examples of dissemination through training exist (Bradshaw *et al.* 2002) and successful models
for service development are available (e.g. Barrowclough *et al.* 1999). Family interventions have advanced from an initial focus on modifying high expressed
emotion in families to a recognition that many families who have a member
diagnosed with schizophrenia will experience a range of disrupting and distressing experiences with which to cope. Offering timely packages that may include
individualised education about all aspects of the illness, stress management,
realistic goal setting, communication skills training and improved problem
solving helps to address some of the difficulties families face.

When we began working with Bob and his family, it became apparent that
unless a family intervention was undertaken, important opportunities would
have been missed in supporting the family and addressing Bob's needs. The
intervention used an eclectic approach based around the cognitive-behavioural
family therapy researched by Barrowclough and Tarrier (1992). It commenced
with giving a detailed rationale for the therapy, which was followed by an in-
depth assessment process. Table 4.5 illustrates the assessment framework.

In summary, the results of the assessments showed a range of needs in a
number of key areas. Feeding back the information from these assessments was
an essential stage in the process of therapy. It incorporated discussion of how
much the family understood about the illness, the distress and restrictions to
lifestyle it had caused, the dissatisfaction with behaviours that had arisen, existing coping strategies and strengths. This is summarised in Table 4.6, which also
briefly illustrates the link between case formulation and intervention.

A range of individualised, targeted interventions that included an education
package, realistic goal setting and stress management (Barrowclough and Tarrier
1992) were agreed in response to the family case formulation. The interventions
were delivered over ten sessions.

Education package

Although education alone appears not to lead to successful outcomes in family
interventions (Tarrier *et al.* 1988), providing information and exploring relatives'
illness models has played a major part in most research studies (Leff *et al.* 1982,
Falloon *et al.* 1982, Barrowclough and Tarrier 1987). The strategy adopted with Bob
and his family drew on the principles of both deficit and interactional models of
information delivery. Deficit models, which concentrate on providing new information to eliminate deficits in knowledge, may result in beneficial changes in
attitudes and behaviours. The interactional model (Barrowclough and Tarrier
1992) allows a removal of context from 'disease' to 'illness'; and a focus on patient's
and relative's own 'illness models'. This approach helps the assimilation and
understanding of new material while maintaining respect for existing beliefs.
Although Barrowclough and Tarrier recommend the interactional model for families who have been living with schizophrenia for many years, as Bob has had a

Table 4.5 Summary of family assessments and rationale for use.

Assessment	Rationale for choice
Relative Assessment Interview (RAI, Barrowclough and Tarrier 1992)	Adapted from the Camberwell Family Interview (Leff 1985). This is a semi-structured interview to gain information from individual family members and requires a conversational style. It can take several sessions to complete and elicits background information pertaining to the family, the mental health history of the client and information about past and current episodes of illness and symptoms. Relationships between members of the family is sought alongside general information about family life, including levels of activity, physical health, interests, employment and social lives. It enhances engagement and can be cathartic in its own right
Knowledge about Schizophrenia Interview (KASI, Barrowclough *et al.* 1987)	This is designed to assess the carer's knowledge, beliefs and attitudes about schizophrenia. It is useful when planning education sessions based on the carers' model of illness and enables the design of an individualised and interactional education package. Completed with each family member individually. A conversational style should be used
General Health Questionnaire (GHQ, Goldberg and Williams 1988)	Validated by the World Health Organization, this assessment measures psychological distress by means of closed self-rating questions. The number of questions depends on the version being used. Different scoring methods are also used which can affect the external validity of the measure
Family Questionnaire (FQ, Barrowclough and Tarrier 1992)	A self-rated checklist of 49 questions rated on a five-point scale. Used to assess for behaviours that carers report as being distressing. The frequency of the behaviour, the amount of distress the behaviour causes and current levels of coping are recorded. It is a reliable and valid tool, useful as a measure of both process and outcome

relatively recent onset of illness, a combination of both models, based on individualised assessment and formulation, was utilised.

Education took place over three sessions. A range of written and video material was utilised. Unusually in the author's experience, Bob's mother provided some of this information from searches online. Bob attended the second of these sessions to allow him to 'tell his own story'. On review of the education package, his parents found hearing about Bob's experiences in detail for the first time the most valuable part of these sessions.

Stress management

Cognitive-behavioural interventions to reduce levels of reported stress are advocated as a continuous process in the delivery of family interventions (Barrowclough and Tarrier 1992). This section of the intervention was directly

Table 4.6 Organisation of family assessment material (family case formulation).

Subject area	Summary of information	'Problems' into 'needs'

Understanding the illness:
  Information primarily gathered from KASI
  Additional material provided by informal discussion
	Mother has researched psychosis and intervention possibilities. Knowledgeable about medication. Can be pessimistic about prognosis
	Father has deficits in knowledge of treatment options, associations between psychosis and stress, medication and negative symptoms
		To engage in an **education package** based on family's understanding of Bob's illness. Shortfalls in knowledge need to be addressed, existing information confirmed as accurate and new information shared.
		Treatment options need to be discussed

Situations triggering distress:
  Assessed via FQ, RAI, COPM and informal discussion
	Main areas causing distress
	  Bob staying in bed and not managing his self-care.
	This causes mother to shout at him, which in turn causes Bob to become upset
		Enhance problem-solving skills to help resolve issues effectively as they arise
		Develop **stress management** strategies

Coping strategies: Assessed via FQ, RAI, COPM, ACI and informal interview	All family members have developed coping strategies to deal with stressful situations. Some of these are more useful and effective than others	Assess adaptive strategies and those that worsen situations Develop alternative strategies to replace maladaptive ones **Goal setting** to practice new strategies
Restrictions to life style: Assessed via RAI and informal interview	Mother and father have experienced significant restrictions to life style	To review restrictions to lifestyle and to rectify deficits involving the use of both **Stress management and goal setting** Interventions
Dissatisfaction with Bob's behaviour: Assessed via FQ, RAI and informal interview	Parents get angry with Bob staying in bed and not taking enough care of his personal needs	To address those behaviours that mum finds difficult – either to modify behaviour OR to help mum to cope better
Strengths	Commitment to coping with illness as well as possible; informed knowledge and interest about the illness; able to work with services	The family need the opportunity to remind themselves of their strengths, skills and positive strategies for coping

For abbreviations see Table 4.5.

related to assessment material via the individualised formulation. The application of stress management principles to address a number of issues directly contributed by family members as important and prioritised by the family has proved to be an effective method to improve relationships within the family. It supports them in becoming more confident of addressing problems as they arise.

An example of the model's effectiveness was the work undertaken to address the issue of Bob and his parents arguing when he refuses to get out of bed in the morning and attend to his personal hygiene needs. The process commenced with a detailed examination of the stressful situation. It became clear that when Bob didn't respond initially to his mum's requests to get out of bed and have a shower, she became angry and upset with him. On one occasion she even burst into his room to shout at him to 'get up, you lazy ***'. Bob then accused his mum of 'trying to control me', while his mum called him 'ungrateful' for all she did for him. They were both left feeling angry and upset. Using a self-monitoring form, both Bob and his mum agreed to record in detail the above incident and other similar occurrences, rating the feelings generated by these incidents using a 1–10 scale. When this form was reviewed at the next meeting, it enabled us to discuss alternative ways of responding when arguments like this arose. Bob suggested that if his mum would give him an initial shout to wake him up, then another call twenty minutes later to remind him, he would then get up and shower if he could. However, he asked his mum not to call him again after this and to trust him to get up if he felt able to. His mum agreed to try this and we discussed different ways she could think about this situation. For instance, it was suggested that as Bob was a grown man now, it was really up to him when he got out of bed. His mum agreed with this and these alternative ways of behaving and thinking about the situation were practised 'in vitro' during the session. New stress monitoring forms were used to compare differences in intensity of feeling before and after the intervention. Evaluation took place after two weeks and minor adjustments could be made at that point.

This method has been adapted to work on other key stressors and is a continuous process necessitating frequent review, evaluation and modification. Not all plans have been successful but the process itself has proved effective and its generalisation to other problem areas is ongoing with this family.

Goal setting

Following the intervention to help manage stress described above, it was important to build on its success by utilising a realistic and achievable goal setting strategy. The emphasis on this section of family intervention is to assess and improve the personal functioning of the patient and to set goals for both the patient and relatives to address wants and needs in areas of quality of life, self-efficacy and independent functioning. We decided to address the issue that had already become evident in earlier sections of the intervention – Bob's self-care, such as getting up, showering, shaving and changing his clothes at least twice a

Table 4.7 Specific example of goal planning.

Key steps in goal setting	Specific intervention techniques
(1) Identification of problem area	Bob and his family have collaboratively identified the problems associated with his current level of functioning in self-care skills
(2) Translate to needs	Re-frame 'problem' using 'constructional approach' – 'if you didn't have this problem/obstacle/deficit what would you be doing instead?' Problem re-framed: 'Bob would like to get up in the mornings and have a shower as he would feel more confident in leaving the house and going to the sports centre and this would also relieve the friction in the house associated with him staying in bed and not washing and changing his clothes.'
(3) Identify strengths	Review strengths and list them from the formulation: His own room to change in privacy His physical fitness The awareness of being able to cope with his self-care in the past Support from parents Finances to buy new clothes
(4) Set a realistic goal – short-term goal leading to eventual long-term goal	Short-term goals: Bob will get up and wash every day before 11 am and change into clean clothes put out by his mother Steps needed to attain first short-term goal Drawing on strengths and use of coping strategies Mother to bring him a cup of coffee and turn on radio prior to him getting up but she will just say good morning rather than ask him to get up

week. Table 4.7 illustrates the general principles of this approach as well as the specifics of this intervention.

This intervention closely overlapped with coping strategy enhancement and stress management. The end results were rewarding for the family and therapists. Setting realistic targets and short-term goals leading to eventual long-term aims established a rhythm to working together, enabling Bob to be more confident in his appearance when he went out. This method has been applied to a range of problems and needs identified by family members. For instance, Bob started to do some gardening for elderly neighbours. This re-established his independence, raised his self-esteem and meant that he structured his time more meaningfully.

Task box 4

▪ List the obstacles that might be encountered if someone in the family home becomes acutely psychotic.
▪ How might an occupational therapist be involved in supporting the family to overcome these obstacles?
▪ How might the occupational therapist encounter difficulties when attempting to implement family interventions?

Evaluation of interventions

The individual interventions we implemented involved the introduction of cognitive, behavioural and sensory coping strategies. This approach to reducing stress and increasing coping strategies was a major component in helping Bob to increase his self-efficacy and reduce the distress levels associated with his voice hearing experiences. Instead of the voices being uncontrollable and all-powerful, Bob was able to prove to himself that he could exercise a measure of control over them. Decreasing his arousal and increasing his ability to distract himself from them replaced the less useful coping strategy of shouting at the voices. However, Bob did continue to prefer to use alcohol instead of taking additional prescribed medication. Bob was able to visit the gym on a regular basis when a friend accompanied him, although he now wants to try to go there alone.

Outcomes were measured once again using the COPM and his scores had increased in the areas of his subjective performance and satisfaction. Bob completed an evaluation of his experience of the occupational therapy interventions and both objective and subjective data were acquired and entered on a database for audit purposes. A summative report was completed and sent to his care team. Bob was discharged from the Home Treatment Team and a referral was made for the occupational therapy in the Community Mental Health Team to offer continued occupational therapist input to facilitate Bob in achieving further goals.

The formal methods for evaluation employed in the family intervention were primarily via re-assessment utilising original family intervention assessment tools. The family questionnaire was repeated to ascertain whether there had been a modification of disturbing behaviours or responses to it. The KASI was repeated at the conclusion of the education package to assess whether there had been any impact on either knowledge about the illness or attributions given to it. The GHQ was repeated with both parents to ascertain whether interventions had affected stress levels or psychological well-being.

On discussion with Bob and his parents, they all agreed that they were more knowledgeable about the illness, better able to identify and cope with stress, set realistic goals and to solve problems as they arose. Bob remains close to both his mum and dad and finds their ongoing support invaluable. He now manages to get up most mornings and changes his clothes regularly. He has grown a beard rather than shaving every day but he does shower at least twice a week. His mother continues to prompt him but she has refrained from getting into arguments with him. Instead, she is supportive when he does manage to cope with his personal care. As Bob is now able to get up earlier, and he is starting to use his time more productively. He has now identified his next goal, which is to build on his interest in gardening.

Conclusion

Owing to the limitations of previous studies, researchers have formulated increasingly stringent methods to evaluate efficacy and develop innovative methods of applying basic principles in the field of psychosis. Interest in psychological interventions for psychosis continues to develop. The efficacy of the interventions will also be able to be more accurately determined as the emergence of increased grant-funded research enables more stringent studies to be conducted. While the literature has informed clinical practice by the provision of working knowledge, psychological treatments for psychotic clients are a scarce resource. Interventions are time consuming and few staff are skilled in their use. Research has not yet addressed issues of resources and service provision (Jones *et al.* 2006). Psychological treatments, however, have the potential to reduce costs by reducing the length of in-patient admissions and delaying relapse (Drury *et al.* 1996).

References

Andreasen, N.C. (1984) *The Scale for the Assessment of Negative Symptoms (SANS)*. Iowa City, IA: The University of Iowa Press.

Baguley, I. and Baguley, C. (1999) Psychosocial interventions in the treatment of psychosis. *Mental Health Care*. **21**: 314–18.

Barrowclough, C. and Tarrier, N. (1992) *Families of Schizophrenic Patients: Cognitive-behavioural interventions*. London: Chapman and Hall.

Barrowclough, C., Tarrier, N., Watts, S., Vaughn, C., Bamrah, J.S. and Freeman, H.L. (1987) Assessing the functional value of relatives' reported knowledge about schizophrenia. *British Journal of Psychiatry*. **151**: 1–8.

Barrowclough, C., Tarrier, N., Lewis, S., Sellwood, W., Mainwaring, J., Quinn, J. and Hamlin, C. (1999) Randomised controlled effectiveness trial of a needs based psychosocial intervention service for carers of people with schizophrenia. *British Journal of Psychiatry*. **174**: 505–11.

Beck, A.T. (1952) Successful outpatient psychotherapy of a chronic schizophrenic with a delusion based on borrowed guilt. *Psychiatry*. **15**: 305–12.

Bentall, R.P. (1996) From cognitive studies of psychosis to cognitive behaviour therapy for psychotic symptoms. In: Haddock, G. and Slade, P.D. (eds) *Cognitive Behavioural Interventions with Psychotic Disorders*. London: Routledge.

Birchwood, M., and MacMillan, J.F. (1993) Early intervention in schizophrenia. *Australian and New Zealand Journal of Psychiatry*. **27**: 374–8.

Birchwood, M., Smith, J., Cochrane, R., Wetton, S. and Copestake, S. (1990) The social functioning scale: The development and validation of a scale of social adjustment for use in family intervention programmes with schizophrenic patients. *British Journal of Psychiatry*. **157**: 853–9.

Birchwood, M., Smith, J., Macmillan, F. and McGovern, D. (1998) Early interventions in psychotic relapse. In: Brooker, C. and Repper, J. (eds) *Serious Mental Health Problems in the Community: Policy, Practice and Research*. London: Baillière Tindall.

Bradshaw, T., Mairs, H. and Lowndes, F. (2002) The COPE initiative: four years on. *Mental Health Nursing*. **23**: 4–6.

Brown, G.W., Birley, J.L.T. and Wing, J.K. (1972) Influence of family life on the course of schizophrenic disorder. *British Journal of Psychiatry*. **121**: 241–58.

Brown, W.A. and Herz, L.R. (1989) Response to neuroleptic drugs as a device for classifying schizophrenia. *Schizophrenia Bulletin*. **15**: 123–9.

Carr, V. (1988) Patients' techniques for coping with schizophrenia: An exploratory study. *British Journal of Medical Psychology*. **61**: 339–52.

Carter, D.M., Mackinnon, A. and Copolov, D.L. (1996) Patients' strategies for coping with auditory hallucinations. *Journal of Nervous and Mental Disease*. **184**: 159–64.

CRD (2001) Undertaking systematic reviews of research on effectiveness: CRD guidance for those carrying out or commissioning reviews – CRD Report Number 4 (2nd edn). Centre for Reviews and Dissemination. Available from: www.york.ac.uk/inst/crd/report4.htm (accessed 03/2004).

Chadwick, P. and Birchwood, M. (1994) The omnipotence of voices I: a cognitive approach to auditory hallucinations. *British Journal of Psychiatry*. **164**: 190–201.

Chadwick, P. and Birchwood, M. (1995) The omnipotence of voices II: The beliefs about voices questionnaire (BAVQ). *British Journal of Psychiatry*. **166**: 190–201.

Chadwick, P., Lees, S. and Birchwood, M. (2000) The revised beliefs about voices questionnaire (BAVQ-R). *British Journal of Psychiatry*. **177**: 229–32.

Chadwick, P.D. and Lowe, C.F. (1990) Measurement and modification of delusional beliefs. *Journal of Consulting and Clinical Psychology*. **58**: 225–32.

Cormac, I., Jones, C., Campbell, C., Silveira de Mota Neto J. (2006) Cognitive-behaviour therapy for schizophrenia. *The Cochrane Library*. Issue 4. Oxford: Update Software.

Curson, D.A., Patel, M. and Liddle P.F. (1988) Psychiatric morbidity of a long term hospital population with chronic schizophrenia and implications for long term community care. *BMJ*. **297**: 819–22.

Crowther, R.E., Marshall, M., Bond, G.R. and Huxley, P. (2001) Helping people with severe mental illness to obtain work: systematic review. *BMJ*. **322**: 204–8.

Deegan, P. (1998) Recovery: the lived experience of rehabilitation. *Psychosocial Rehabilitation Journal*. **11**: 11–19.

DoH (1990) *Caring for People – Community Care in the Next Decade and Beyond*. London, HMSO.

Dittman, J. and Schüttler, R. (1990) Disease consciousness and coping strategies of patients with schizophrenic psychosis. *Acta Psychiatrica Scandinavica*. **82**: 318–22.

Drury, V., Birchwood, M., Cochrane, R. and MacMillan, F. (1996) Cognitive behaviour therapy and recovery from acute psychosis: A controlled trial **1**: Impact on psychotic symptoms. *British Journal of Psychiatry*. **169**: 599–612.

Fadden, G. (1997) Implementation of family interventions in routine clinical practice following staff training programmes: A major cause for concern. *Journal of Mental Health.* **6**: 599–612.

Fadden, G. (1998) Family intervention. In: Brooker, C. and Repper, J. (eds) *Serious Mental Health Problems in the Community: Policy, Practice and Research.* London: Baillière Tindall.

Falloon, I. (ed.) (1985) *Family Management of Schizophrenia.* Baltimore: Johns Hopkins Press.

Falloon, I.R. and Talbot, R.E. (1991) Persistent auditory hallucinations: coping mechanisms and implications for management. *Psychological Medicine.* **11**: 329–39.

Falloon, I.R.H., Boyd, J.L., McGill, C.W., Razani, J., Moss, M.B. and Gilderman, A.M. (1982) Family management in the prevention of exacerbations of schizophrenia: A controlled study. *New England Journal of Medicine.* **306**: 1437–40.

Falloon, I.R.H., Boyd, J.L., McGill, C.W., Williamson, M., Razani, J., Moss, H.B., Gilderman, A.M. and Simson, G.M. (1985) Family management in the prevention of morbidity in schizophrenia: Clinical outcome of a 2 year longitudinal study. *Archives of General Psychiatry.* **42**: 887–96.

Falloon, I.R.H., Rapporta, M., Fadden, G. and Graham-Hole, V. (1993) *Managing Stress in Families: Cognitive and Behavioural Strategies for Enhancing Coping Skills.* London, Routledge.

Finn, S.E., Bailey, J.M. and Schultz, R.T. (1990) Subjective utility ratings of neuroleptics in treating schizophrenia. *Psychological Medicine.* **20**: 843–8.

Fowler, D. and Morley, S. (1989) The cognitive behavioural treatment of hallucinations and delusions: a preliminary study. *Behavioural Psychotherapy.* **58**: 25–34.

Fowles, D.C. (1992) Schizophrenia: diathesis-stress revised. *Annual Review of Psychology.* **43**: 303–6.

Gamble, C. and Brennan, G. (2000) Assessments: A rationale for choosing and learning. In: Gamble, C. and Brennan, G. (eds) *Working with Serious Mental Illness: A Manual for Clinical Practice.* Edinburgh: Elsevier.

Glasziou, P., Irwig, L., Bain, C. and Colditz, G. (2001) *Systematic Reviews in Health Care. A Practical Guide.* Cambridge: Cambridge University Press.

Goldberg, D. and Williams, P. (1988) *A User's Guide to the General Health Questionnaire.* Windsor: NFER-Nelson.

Green, M.F., Hugdahl, K. and Mitchell, S. (1994) Dichotic listening during auditory hallucinations in patients with schizophrenia. *American Journal of Psychiatry.* **151**: 357–62.

Green, P. and Preston, M. (1981) Reinforcement of vocal correlates of auditory hallucinations by auditory feedback: a case study. *British Journal of Psychiatry.* **139**: 204–8.

Haddock G., Bentall, R.P. and Slade, P. (1993) Psychological treatment of chronic auditory hallucinations: Two case studies. *Behavioural and Cognitive Psychotherapy.* **21**: 335–46.

Haddock, G., Slade, P.D., Bentall R.P., Reid, D. and Farager B.F. (1998) A comparison of long term effectiveness of distraction and focusing in the treatment of auditory hallucinations. *British Journal of Medical Psychology.* **71**: 339–49.

Haddock, G., McCarron, J., Tarrier, N. and Farragher, E.B. (1999) Scales to measure dimensions of hallucinations and delusions: The psychotic symptoms rating scales (PSYRATS). *Psychological Medicine.* **29**: 879–89.

Herz, M.I., Lamberti, S., Mintz, J., Scott, R., O'Dell, S.P., McCartan, L. and Nix, G. (2000) A programme for relapse prevention in schizophrenia. *Archives of General Psychiatry.* **57**: 177–283.

Hogarty, G.E., Anderson, C.M., Reiss, D.J., Kornblith, S.J., Greenwald, D.P., Javana, C.D., Madonia, M.J. (1986) Family psychoeducation, social skills training and maintenance chemotherapy in the aftercare treatment of schizophrenia: I. One year effects of a controlled study on relapse and expressed emotion. *Archives of General Psychiatry.* **43**: 633–42.

Hogg, L. (1996) Psychological treatments for negative symptoms. In: Haddock, G. and Slade, P.D. (eds) *Cognitive Behavioural Interventions with Psychotic Disorders.* London: Routledge, pp. 151–67.

Johannessen, J.O. (2001). Early recognition and intervention: The key to success in the treatment of schizophrenia? *Disease Management and Health Outcomes* **9**: 317–27.

Johnstone, E.C., Owens, D.G.C., Gold, A., Crow, T.J. and Macmillan, J.E. (1984) Schizophrenic patients discharged from hospital: a follow-up study. *British Journal of Psychiatry.* **145**: 586–90.

Jones, C., Cormac I., Mota J., Campbell C. (2006) Cognitive behavioural therapy for schizophrenia. *The Cochrane Library.* Issue 3. Oxford: Update Software.

Kane, J.M. (1985) Compliance issues in out-patient treatment. *Journal of Clinical Psychopharmacology.* **5**: 22S–27S.

Kemp, R., Hayward, P., Applewhaite, G., Everitt, B. and David, A. (1996) Compliance therapy in psychotic patients: Randomised controlled trial. *BMJ* **312**: 345–9.

Khan, K.S., Kunz, R., Klieijen, J. and Antes, S. (2003) *Systematic Reviews to Support Evidence Based Medicine: How to Review and Apply Findings of Healthcare Research.* London: Royal Society of Medicine Press.

Kingdon, D. and Turkington, D. (1994) *Cognitive-Behavioural Therapy of Schizophrenia.* Hove: Lawrence Erlbaum Associates.

Krawiecka, M., Goldberg, D. and Vaughan, M. (1977) A standardised psychiatric assessment scale for rating chronic psychiatric patients. *Acta Psychiatrica Scandinavica* **55**: 299–308. Modified by S. Lancashire (1998), University of Manchester, unpublished.

Kuipers, E., Garety, P., Fowler, D., Dunn, D., Freeman, D., Bebbington, P. and Hadley, C. (1997) London and East Anglia randomised controlled trial of cognitive-behavioural therapy for psychosis: Effects of the treatment phase. *British Journal of Psychiatry.* **171**: 319–27.

Kuipers, L. and Bebbington, P. (1985) Relatives as a resource in the management of functional illness. *British Journal of Psychiatry.* **147**: 465–70.

Law, M., Baptiste, S., McColl, M., Opzoomer., A., Polatajko H. and Pollock, N. (1990) Canadian Occupational Performance Measure: An outcome measure for Occupational Therapy. *Canadian Journal of Occupational Therapy.* **57**: 82–7.

Law, M., Baptiste, S., Carswell-Opzoomer, A., McColl, M., Polatajko, H. and Pollock, N. (1991) *Canadian Occupational Performance Measure Manual* (Ist edn.). Toronto: CAOT Publications, ACE.

Law, M., Baptiste, S., Carswell, A., McColl, M., Polatajko, H. and Pollock, N. (1994) *Canadian Occupational Performance Measure* (2nd edn.). Montreal: CAOT Publications.

Leff, J., Kuipers, L., Berkovitz, R., Eberlein-Vries, R. and Sturgeon, D. (1982) A controlled trial of social intervention in the families of schizophrenic patients. *British Journal of Psychiatry.* **141**: 121–34.

Leff, J., Kuipers, L., Berkovitz, R. and Sturgeon, D. (1985) A controlled trial of social intervention in the families of schizophrenic patients: Two-year follow-up. *British Journal of Psychiatry.* **146**: 594–600.

Lehman, A.F., Steinwachs, D.M., and the Co-Investigators of the PORT Project (1998) At Issue: Translating research into practice: The Schizophrenia Patient Outcomes Research Team (PORT) treatment recommendations. *Schizophrenia Bulletin.* **24**: 1–10.

Lindsley, O.R. (1959) Reduction in rate of vocal psychotic symptoms by differential positive reinforcement. *Journal of the Experimental Analysis of Behaviour.* **2**: 269.

Margo, A., Hemsley, D.R. and Slade, P.D. (1981) The effects of varying auditory input on schizophrenic hallucinations. *British Journal of Psychiatry.* **39**: 101–7.

Marshall, M., Lockwood, A., Gray, A., *et al.* (2006) Assertive community treatment for people with severe mental disorders. In: Schizophrenia Module of the *Cochrane Database Systematic Reviews.* Oxford: Update Software.

Marwaha, S. and Johnson, S. (2005) Views and experiences of employment among people with psychosis: a qualitative descriptive study. *International Journal of Social Psychiatry.* **51**: 302–16.

Milton, F., Patwa, V.K. and Hafner, R.J. (1978) Confrontation versus belief modification in persistently deluded patients. *British Journal of Medical Psychology.* **51**: 127–30.

Morrison, A.P., French, P., Walford, L., Lewis, S.W., Kilcommons, A., Green, J., Parker, S. and Bentall, R.P. (2004) Cognitive therapy for the prevention of psychosis in people at ultra-high risk: Randomisd controlled trial. *British Journal of Psychiatry.* **185**: 291–7.

Murphy, E., Dingwall, R., Greatbatch, D., Parker, S. and Watson, P. (1998) Qualitative research methods in health technology assessment: a review of the literature. Southampton National Co-ordinating Centre for Health Technology Assessment. Available from: http://www.hta.nhsweb.nhs.uk/ (accessed on 16/02/2005).

Mueser, K., Drake, R. and Bond, G. (1997) Recent advances in psychiatric rehabilitation for patients with severe mental illness. *Harvard Review of Psychiatry.* **5**: 123–37.

Nelson, H.E., Thrasher, S. and Barnes, T.R.E. (1991) Practical ways of alleviating auditory hallucinations. *BMJ.* 302–327.

National Institute for Clinical Excellence (2002) *Schizophrenia: Core Interventions in the Treatment and Management of Schizophrenia in Primary and Secondary Care.* London: National Institute of Clinical Excellence.

Nuechterlein, K.H. and Dawson, M.E. (1984) A heuristic vulnerability-stress model of schizophrenic episodes. *Schizophrenia Bulletin.* **10**: 300–12.

Nydegger, R.V. (1972) The elimination of hallucinatory and delusional behaviour by verbal conditioning and assertive training: A case study. *Journal of Behaviour Therapy and Experimental Psychiatry.* **3**: 225–7.

Oliver, J.P., Huxley, P.J., Priebe, S. and Kaiser, W. (1997) Measuring the quality of life of severely mentally ill people using the Lancashire Quality of Life Profile. *Social Psychiatry and Epidemiology.* **32**: 76–83.

Overall, J.E. and Gorham, D.R. (1962) The Brief Psychiatric Rating Scale. *Psychological Reports.* **10**: 799–812.

Pekkala, E. and Merinder, L. (2006) Psychoeducation for Schizophrenia. *The Cochrane Database of Systematic Reviews.* Issue 2. Oxford: Update Software.

Pharoah, F.M., Mari, J.J. and Streiner, D. (2006) Family intervention for schizophrenia. *The Cochrane Library.* Issue 3. Oxford Update Software.

Pilling, S., Bebbington, P. and Kuipers, E. (2002) Psychological treatments in schizophrenia: I. Meta-analysis of family intervention and cognitive-behaviour therapy. *Psychological Medicine.* **32**: 763–82.

Popay, J. and Williams, G. (1998) Qualitative research and evidence based healthcare. *Journal of Research Sociology and Medicine.* **86**: 91–5.

Rebeiro, K. (1998) Occupation as means to mental health: A review of the literature and a call for research. *Canadian Journal of Occupational Therapy.* **65**: 12–19.

Robertson, L., Connaughton, J.A. and Nicol, M.M. (2006) Life skills programmes for chronic mental illnesses. *The Cochrane Library.* Issue 2. Oxford: Update Software.

Rollnick, S. and Miller, W.R. (1995) What is motivational interviewing? *Behavioural and Cognitive Psychotherapy* **23**: 325–34.

Romme, M.A. and Escher, S. (1989) Hearing voices. *Schizophrenia Bulletin* **15**: 209–16.

Rosenburg, M. (1965) *Society and the Adolescent Self-image.* New York: Princeton University Press.

Rossler, W., Loffler, W., Fatkenheuer, B. and Riecher-Rossler, A. (1995) Case management for schizophrenic patients at risk for rehospitalization: a case control study. *European Archives of Psychiatry and Clinical Neuroscience.* **246**: 29–36.

Ryrie, I. (2000) Assessing risk. In: Gamble, C. and Brennan G. (eds) *Working with Serious Mental Illness: A Manual for Clinical Practice.* Edinburgh: Bailliere Tindall.

Sensky, T., Turkington, D., Kingdon, D., Scott, J., Scott, J., Siddle, R., O'Carroll, M. and Barnes, T. (2000) A randomised controlled trial of CBT for persistent symptoms of schizophrenia resistant to medication. *Archives of General Psychiatry.* **57**: 165–72.

Tarrier, N. (1987) An investigation of residual psychotic symptoms in discharged schizophrenic patients. *British Journal of Clinical Psychology.* **26**: 141–3.

Tarrier, N. (2002) The use of coping strategies and self-regulation in the treatment of psychosis. In: Morrison, A.P. (ed.) *A Casebook of Cognitive Therapy for Psychosis.* Hove: Brunner-Routledge.

Tarrier, N., Barrowclough, C., Vaughn, C., Bamrah, J.S., Pordeccu, K., Watts, S. and Freeman, H. (1988) The community management of schizophrenia: A controlled trial of a behavioural intervention with families to reduce relapse. *British Journal of Psychiatry.* **165**: 532–42.

Tarrier, N., Barrowclough, C., Vaughn, C., Bamrah, J.S., Pordeccu, K., Watts, S. and Freeman, H. (1989) Community management of schizophrenia: A two-year follow-up of a behavioural intervention with families. *British Journal of Psychiatry.* **154**: 625–8.

Tarrier, N., Beckett, R., Harwood, S., Baker, A., Yusupoff, L. and Ugarteguru, I. (1993) A controlled trial of two cognitive-behavioural methods of treating drug-resistant residual symptoms in schizophrenic patients: 1. Outcome. *British Journal of Psychiatry.* **162**: 524–32.

Tarrier, N., Yusupoff, L., Kinney, C., McCarthy, E., Gledhill, A., Haddock, G. and Morris, J. (1998) Randomised controlled trial intensive cognitive-behavioural therapy for patients with chronic schizophrenia. *BMJ.* **317**: 303–7.

Tarrier, N., Wittkowski, A., Kinney, C., McCarthy, E., Morris, J. and Humphreys, L. (1999) Durability of the effects of cognitive-behavioural therapy in the treatment of chronic schizophrenia: 12-month follow-up. *British Journal of Psychiatry.* **174**: 500–4.

Tarrier, N., Lewis, S., Haddock, G., Bentall, R., Drake, R., Kinderman, P., Kingdon, D., Siddle, R., Everitt, J., Leadley, K., Benn, A., Grazebrook, K., Haley, C., Akhtar, S., Davies, L., Palmer, A. and Dunn, G. (2004) Cognitive-behavioural therapy in first-episode and early schizophrenia. *British Journal of Psychiatry*. **184**: 231–9.

Vaughn, C. and Leff, J. (1976) The influence of family and social factors on the course of psychiatric illness. *British Journal of Psychiatry*. **129**: 125–37.

Watts, F.N., Powell, G.E. and Austin, S.V. (1973) The modification of abnormal beliefs. *British Journal of Medical Psychology*. **46**: 359–63.

World Schizophrenia Fellowship (1997) Strategy development: Family interventions work: Putting research findings into practice. Report of the World Schizophrenia Fellowship, following discussions at the Christchurch Convention Centre, New Zealand, September 4–5.

Wykes, T., Reeder, C., Williams, C., Corner, J., Rice, C. and Everitt, B. (2003) Are the effects of cognitive remediation therapy (CRT) durable? Results from an exploratory trial. *Schizophrenia Research*. **61**: 163–74.

Zubin, J. and Spring, B. (1977) Vulnerability – a new view on schizophrenia. *Journal of Abnormal Psychology*. **86**: 103–26.

5: Not drowning but waving: working with female survivors of childhood sexual abuse

Cathy Long

Childhood sexual abuse (CSA) is an emotive and inevitably uncomfortable issue for everyone, as it crosses all boundaries of cultural norms and goes against what is morally and socially accepted behaviour towards children. The widely publicised access to web-based pornographic material involving children has brought CSA once again into the public arena. CSA comes in many different guises as will be briefly discussed but regardless of form, it occurs in all strata of society – rich or poor and any occupational, ethnic or religious group (Holz 1994). It is still a taboo subject, but loosening of taboos about sexual activity generally may have affected both the incidence and levels of reporting of CSA.

CSA has received little attention in occupational therapy literature yet research consistently finds that survivors of childhood sexual abuse have more health-related problems than do the general population (Hulme and Grove 1994, Holz 1994, Creedy, *et al.* 1998, Griffiths 1998, Monahan and Forgash 2000, Schachter *et al.* 2004). More specifically statistical evidence suggests women using mental health services are more likely to have experienced CSA than women attending general practices (Palmer *et al.* 1993). In general, there is consensus in the literature of a higher incidence of CSA among women receiving professional help for problems of a psycho-social nature, with some research suggesting that as many as a quarter of all women in the USA were subjected to CSA (Finkelhor *et al.* 1990, cited by Hall and Kondora 1997).

This chapter will first introduce some of the possible health and psycho-social consequences of CSA; second it will present guiding principles for occupational therapy practice and intervention by referring to the literature in this field; and finally it will present 'Karen' to show one way of implementing occupational therapy process in more detail. My aim is not to prepare you to work with a client specifically on the experience of the abuse itself – this is skilled work and if poorly and insensitively executed can add to the trauma rather than heal and help. The Code of Ethics and Professional Conduct (College of Occupational Therapists (COT) 2005) requires us to practice within our professional competence and to only provide services for which we are qualified or experienced. I hope however that you will learn something more about CSA and what constitutes good practice when working as an occupational therapist with someone who has a history of CSA. In this way, client-centred practice for women who have been abused might be enhanced.

Some statistics

The women's mental health strategy (Department of Health (DoH) 2002) states that studies reveal women are three times more likely to have been abused than men, with men consistently being the perpetrators of abuse in 95% of cases for both abused boys and girls. Intra-familial abuse (incest) is more common in girls (DoH 2002) and according to Meekums (2000) previously known and trusted males (fathers, brothers, stepfathers, baby sitters, priests, teachers, therapists) tend to be the perpetrators of CSA more than strangers.

Defining CSA

Russell's definition of CSA is commonly referred to throughout literature: as any sexualised behaviour between an adolescent, adult or older sibling and a younger child (Russell 1986). According to Bohn and Holz (1996) sexually exploitative behaviour might range from lewd and lascivious behaviour (e.g. showing pornographic material, exposing genitalia) to more aggressive sexual behaviours (digital or object penetration, oral sex and sexual intercourse).

Dynamics of CSA

According to Herman (1992) secrecy, betrayal, isolation and stigmatisation are typical features of CSA. Issues of power, control and authority are also significant and often lead to feelings of anxiety in the context of treatment (Monahan and Forgash 2000). The aim of this section is to introduce theoretical perspectives which help to explain why these phenomena are associated with CSA.

Family systems theory

First, literature underlines possible issues with control, as the experience of abuse involves a child being physically and mentally overpowered by a sometimes previously trusted adult. Finkelhor (1982) has written extensively about CSA and suggests that it flourishes in particular circumstances which tend to increase the risk of CSA: high degree of family isolation; a dominating father who can do what he wants with his children; and children exposed to an increased number of stepfathers or mothers' boyfriends and lovers.

Further theories describe the process of development of an incestuous family, which over time becomes more closed and rigid – outwardly appearing traditional and protective while inwardly being governed by the patriarch. Initially abuse may occur as the child is unquestioningly trusting of the authority figure; later as the child reaches adolescence threats of violence might be necessary to preserve secrecy. Secret promises or special gifts might be other means used by the perpetrator to maintain control over the relationship with the child. A major deterrent of CSA is the presence of a protective mother – in incestuous families this role is not fulfilled. The mother may try to protect the child but eventually succumbs to ignoring or sometimes abetting the abuse. The long-term effect of this betrayal of relationship between child and primary caregiver is thought to have potentially major implications for the child's future mental health and well-being (Coker 1990).

Feminist theory

The women's movement of the 1970s and 1980s broke the silence that generally shrouded violence towards women and children, and in relation to CSA helped to turn over the legacy left by Freud (CSA was considered to be fantasy rather than having any basis in reality – its existence was thus denied) (Hall and Kondora 1997).

The importance of the context of women's lives is underlined in feminist psycho-social theory and an important part of this is the effect of power imbalance and social inequality based on gender. Williams (2005) proposes that CSA (and all other forms of abuse) is a serious abuse of power which is underpinned by the belief that men should have their needs met by women and that these take precedence over the needs of women. Characteristics associated with masculinity (independence; goal attainment; emotional inexpression) all contribute to this belief and serve to distance men from their own and others' emotions, and the emotional consequences of their acts. Thus gender inequalities serve to oppress both men and women.

Creedy *et al.* (1998) drawing on theories of Miller (1976) and Gilligan (1982) propose that women gain strength through their relationships with others; that women's lives and their sense of self are intrinsically linked to and shaped by others. Setting this in a context where the leading valued goals are autonomy, personal achievement and independence the need for connectedness to others and their environment is seen as a weakness rather than a strength.

Creedy *et al.* outlined a framework for working with women survivors of CSA, based on self-in-relation theory which values partnership as the basis for change and proposes that women's psychological distress is exacerbated by their lack of control over what is valued by society.

False memory syndrome

Hall and Kondora (1997) outline and question this notion. Supporters of false memory syndrome accuse therapists of naively accepting everything clients put before them or of planting memories of abuse – as a means of explaining their difficulties. This accusation is especially likely where clients have suppressed painful memories. Hall and Kondora suggest that the support for false memory syndrome is fuelled by society's wish to deny CSA because its existence 'fractures cultural values about families'. One of the consequences for survivors of suppressing memories is the gaps it leaves in a person's history – for some people this can mean feeling dislocated from their pasts.

Coping strategies

Some of the effects listed below are more usefully considered to be coping strategies by some authors. Griffiths (1998), for example, identifies self-harming behaviours, use of drugs and alcohol and suicide as ways of coping with the abuse rather than these being effects of it. Making cuts to arms or other parts of the body might be an attempt to deal with the emotional pain and this need not all be based on negative experiences of CSA. For example feelings of guilt are especially common if the survivor found the experience of CSA pleasurable.

Sequelae of CSA

For some women the abuse experience might have been so traumatising that it has been pushed out of their awareness (Hall and Kondora 1997) and it is only in adulthood that memories are triggered leading to anxiety, panic and flashbacks to the abuse. However, the physical, psychological and sexual effects can be far-reaching and are well documented throughout literature. There is some suggestion that effects are influenced by specific characteristics of the abuse, family dynamics and the survivor. For example, a quantitative study by Hulme and Grove (1994) found a correlation between the duration of the abuse and the number of psycho-social effects. Physical symptoms and effects might include: chronic pelvic pain; gastro-intestinal disorders; epilepsy; irritable bowel syndrome; and persistent headaches (Sheldon 1998). A wide range of somatic symptoms without any physical cause are also common (Holz 1994). Psycho-social symptoms and effects might include: post-traumatic stress; self-injury; helplessness; hopelessness; de-personalisation; paralysis of initiative; repeated search for a rescuer; persistent distrust; depression; fearful of loss of control; shame; embarrassment; lack of trust; sleep disturbance and anxiety (Monahan and Forgash 2000). Low self-esteem, anger and guilt are also common features (Griffiths 1998). Women may present with a personality disorder and/or an eating disorder and might abuse alcohol or drugs (Sheldon 1998). Psychosexual dysfunction might also be a feature.

It is also important to note that CSA may occur in a range of other problems and behaviours, for example, alcohol/drug or physical abuse and it could be dangerous to assume all problems are a direct consequence of CSA. Furthermore some of the sequelae mentioned above could also be described as coping strategies albeit ones that could have detrimental effects on health.

CSA does not necessarily lead to impaired function in later life as there are also some women who have been abused who do not experience any long-term health effects. Binder *et al.* (1996) focused on this group of women and documented circumstances which seemed to protect them from longer-term effects. These included: shorter duration of abuse; absence of physical force; having a supportive and loving person in the environment; perpetrator who was a non-relative; the victim of CSA having special talents or abilities which enabled her to get through the abuse. Having the motivation to leave the abusive situation as soon as possible and being able to see that the perpetrator was evil (thereby externalising the abuse) were also significant protectors.

General issues for practice

The ways in which a person who has been sexually abused presents varies: CSA victims may present as compliant; passive non-resistant; or oppositional and defiant (Monahan and Forgash 2000). However, literature is unanimous in establishing the ways in which clinical practice can be more sensitive to the needs of women who have experienced sexual abuse (Glaister and Abel 2001, Monahan and Forgash 2000, Schachter *et al.* 2004). Some of these recommendations underpin all good mental health practice and are congruent with all client-centred occupational therapy – for example, the importance of a trusting, consistent relationship with a therapist who works within the limitations of their knowledge and capability. (Consideration of the issues for health professions working with this client group are discussed on page 91.)

However, as outlined above, a range of specific issues for survivors of CSA affect practice, and inevitably there is no one approach that will fit all. These are general principles, some of which are supported by research evidence, while others are based upon authors' clinical experience and client testimony. Issues of disclosure of sexual abuse are touched upon on page 84 as this demands extra attention.

▪ *A way of being.* Respectful, consistent, validating and believing of person's story (Abraham 1998). Listening without 'over identification' (Krenken and van Stolk 1990) and with calmness, concern and compassion (Schachter *et al.* 2004) are important conditions for a trusting relationship. According to Monahan and Forgash (2000), establishing this tone of interaction is more important than asking the right questions.

▪ *Sensitivity and safety.* Includes consistency within the therapeutic relationship, but also requires health professionals to: be vigilant about touch as it is often experienced as invasive (Monahan and Forgash 2000); have an awareness of their own personal boundaries (Wolf 1998); be able to handle issues of confidentiality and referral to other agencies without engendering feelings of betrayal or punishment (Long and Smyth 1998); and finally provide an adequately private environment.

▪ *Issues of power and control.* Wolf (1998) writing from her personal experience of psychotherapy valued the opportunity to set her own limits, at her own pace and being able to create her own healthy personal boundaries. Encouraging such partnership working through sharing and negotiating control and information is important as means of the person 'taking back' control and care of herself. Abraham (1998) suggests fostering control is especially important for women who demonstrate ambivalence towards therapy and might take flight.

▪ *Collaborative practice.* All authors in this area mention the need to co-ordinate care and to work with agencies and health care professionals to ensure women's physical, social and psychological needs are addressed. However, careful attention to confidentiality is required, for example discussing with clients the need to share certain pieces of information and to gain her consent to do so (Monahan and Forgash 2000). Although their article focuses on mental health practice, it highlights particular difficulties for women in managing their physical health care. For example, women may fear physical examinations or due to feelings of depression have neglected to seek help for medical problems. This is an important area and occupational therapists in some settings may have a role in supporting women with medical appointments.

For further information see further reading at the end of the chapter.

Responding to disclosure of CSA

Disclosing sexual abuse is difficult for all concerned and there is no right way to facilitate disclosure of CSA. But generally a woman is unlikely to disclose if unsure about how the information will be received (Schachter *et al.* 2004) For example if she thinks she might not be believed or if the therapist responds in an over-intense manner she is less likely to disclose – so the same principles of calmness and concern apply. Generally screening for CSA takes experience but providing the right conditions for a trusting relationship might make a woman feel safe enough to disclose sexual abuse at times when it is unexpected. In this situation, measuring our responses and those of the client is important as is not straying out of professional and personal limits of knowledge or experience. Sensitive discussion of referral to another service or professional might be necessary – prior knowledge of such services is helpful but may not always be possible. For obvious reasons, following through on any promises made is essential.

Task box 1

Given that CSA is emotive and clients who have been abused can be sensitive to the responses of therapists it would be useful to try to think how you might feel if a client disclosed that they had been abused. As you read through think about how these principles might help you to respond effectively.

Theory into practice

Introducing Karen

Karen is 20 years old. She lives on her own in a one-bedroomed flat in a small market town in England. She feels she has done very little with her life until now except for making 'a bit of a mess of it'. She is currently attending a psychiatric day hospital and has been for the past 5 weeks, after becoming increasingly depressed and anxious following the breakdown of her relationship with Jon.

Significant historical events

Karen left school at 16, with five GCSEs and having gained qualifications in computer skills she got a temporary job at a firm of solicitors. Shortly after this she left the family home to live with her boyfriend Jon. Two years later when Karen was pregnant, she experienced flashbacks and feelings of extreme panic during a medical examination. Shortly afterwards she started to make superficial cuts to her inner arms and thighs. Rows between Karen and Jon were increasingly common and both were finding it difficult to cope. Three months into her pregnancy, Karen lost the baby due to a miscarriage and suddenly found that she was very isolated from her family and friends and although she continued to live with Jon, the relationship was very strained. Karen had had periods of depression since she was 17 and although she had responded reasonably well to anti-depressants, this was 'the last straw'.

Karen was admitted to the psychiatric inpatient ward under section 2 of the Mental Health Act (1983) following a serious overdose. She was diagnosed as having post-traumatic stress disorder and depression and prescribed medication to help alleviate the symptoms – she responded well to both this and the hospital environment. However, concerns were expressed that Karen could become overly dependent on the ward, so the team and Karen worked towards discharge to a new flat. After she was discharged Karen continued to experience feelings of anxiety, panic and hopelessness. Karen was referred to the psychiatric day hospital for further assessment and intervention.

Introducing the mental health setting and service

The psychiatric day hospital provides specific and individually tailored intervention programmes for people with a range of mental health problems. This usually involved a full assessment of need: medical; financial; employment; education; daily living; risk and safety (including experience of violence and abuse); social; support; coping strategies/resources and carer's needs. From this assessment a care plan is devised by the key worker and in line with the *National Service Framework for Mental Health* (1999) – the care plan also aims to build upon a person's strengths. Examples of interventions include: anxiety management; daily living skills; creative activity; social support; goal setting; vocational rehabilitation; carers support; cognitive behavioural therapy; creative therapies; and solution focused counselling.

The unit follows a multi-disciplinary approach in order to maximise skills and meet client needs more effectively and supportively. The team comprises nursing; medical; psychology; social worker and occupational therapists in additional to support staff. And where possible the team uses National Institute for Health and Clinical Excellence (NICE) guidelines to support and inform their practice, e.g. the guideline for depression (NICE 2004).

Karen agreed to individual cognitive-behavioural therapy sessions with the clinical psychologist. In addition she attended the day hospital three days per week. Initially she attended an open creative writing group and an art group, with the aim to give an outlet to her creativity as she had expressed an interest in artistic pursuits.

Outwardly Karen appeared quiet but compliant with day hospital staff and she made some friends with other people attending the unit. Again she appeared to settle quickly and described feeling less panicky both at home and with other people. Staff on the in-patient ward had said how she appeared contained on the ward and didn't outwardly appear to have any problems or experience any distress – Karen presented in a similar way at the day hospital. She appeared open about her past although it was evident that she had little contact with her family and few friends. Jon had 'disappeared from the scene'.

Needs and strengths as identified by multi-disciplinary team (MDT)

Following a period of MDT assessment Karen and the team identified her needs and strengths (see Table 5.1).

Risk assessment and management

Specific events from Karen's past were documented as follows:

- Suicide attempt, including a description of the events leading up to it. Karen no longer expressing suicidal thoughts but her situation required monitoring by all the psychiatric day hospital staff.

Table 5.1 Karen's needs and strengths.

Needs	Strengths
To develop awareness of thoughts and how these influence her feelings and behaviours	Verbally Karen was unable or unwilling to identify strengths but felt some pride in her educational achievements and employment experience
To develop a broader range of coping strategies and to prevent future relapse	The team identified her ability to get along with others – especially other female clients
To continue taking anti-depressant medication and monitor side-effects	Karen has had periods when she functioned well
To develop support networks in the community	
To consider daily living and future employment needs	

- Self-harm, specifically superficial cuts to inner arms and thighs. Karen reported that she was no longer cutting herself, but again this required monitoring. Karen was encouraged to talk to staff should she feel the urge to cut herself.
- Isolation, social exclusion and occupational alienation. Karen had few social support or leisure interests, feared going out and was currently unemployed. Admission to psychiatric day hospital to further assess needs in this area.
- Recurrent depression and possible over dependency on psychiatric services. Develop a time limited, negotiated and goal-orientated intervention programme.

Karen's developing story

During an individual session with the clinical psychologist, Lisa, Karen disclosed that she had been sexually abused as a child by her father from the age of 7 to 12 years. She had tried to tell someone once before when she was 17, her younger sister Shelley, who had become so incensed by it that she had stopped all communication with Karen. Karen continued to have 1:1 sessions with Lisa, a process of helping her to talk through the experience of abuse and to become more aware of her thoughts and how these were affecting her behaviour and feelings towards herself and others. To think about how she is being affected now and to learn to put the blame for the abuse where it belonged.

Eventually Karen felt more able to start to think realistically and holistically about her future and what she wanted from it. At this point with Karen's agreement she was referred to Claire, the occupational therapist.

Task box 2

There are signs in Karen's story so far which might suggest a history of sexual abuse. Can you identify them?

Occupational therapy

Occupational therapy began after Karen had been seeing the clinical psychologist for two months and was developing a sense of a more hopeful future that she could be a part of and have some influence over. However, she also experienced darker times and had hours in the flat which she struggled to fill in any meaningful way. Karen was experiencing problems with coping on her own, she found evenings and days when she was not at the unit empty and dissatisfying. She identified that although the depression was lifting she did not know what to do and was worried that her resolve would begin to drift. Cognitive strategies helped her with this (e.g. thought stopping and re-framing negative thoughts) but some more practical help was indicated. Karen had met Claire informally in the unit and agreed to her involvement.

Choice of occupational therapy model and implications for Karen

A series of occupational therapy models could have proved helpful to Karen and the occupational therapist. But taking heed of the importance of the issues of control and authority in the therapy, Claire decided upon the Kawa (river) model (Iwama 2005).

The Kawa (river) model was developed by Japanese and Japanese-Canadian occupational therapists in response to professional mandates which 'confounded or ran counter to their clients' culture or world of everyday meanings' (Iwama 2005 p. 214). The model is derived from Eastern philosophy which purports that the individual is in balance with their surrounding environment and it is this harmony with everyone and everything around that provides energy for life. Thus successful co-existence within a person's contextual environment is what is important to healthy living. This contrasts with a Western ideal which emphasises individual determinism, autonomy, personal independence and freedom.

The Kawa model is devoid of rigid, explicit and universal postulates and is concerned with subjective experience. It is a model potentially rich in imagery and is open to alteration by therapists in both concept and structure, so is able to match specific social and cultural contexts of clients. It is on this basis that I have presented it here – despite its apparent lack of qualitative or scientific underpinning – as a useful tool when working with Karen. The model provides a means of better understanding the complex occupational worlds of clients. A brief description of the model as described by Michael Iwama (2005) follows.

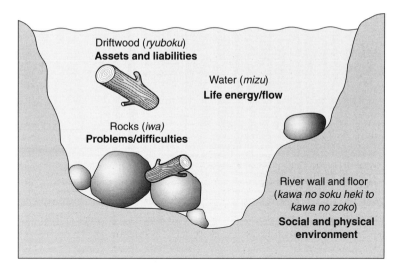

Figure 5.1 The Kawa model. Redrawn from *Occupational Therapy Without Borders*, Kronenberg, F., p.1 © 2004, with permission from Elsevier.

Structure of the Kawa (river) model

The model uses the river (in Japanese *kawa*) as a metaphor for visually describing aspects of the self and one's context over the passage of time. It supposes that life is like a river flowing from birth to death, and in the river are obstacles (rocks (*iwa*)) and driftwood (assets and liabilities (*ryuboku*)) that affect the flow of the river (Figure 5.1). In the river is of course water (*mizu*) which represents life flow or energy for life – the water connects all the elements of the model together, which in harmony with Japanese culture, places much greater value on relationships, belonging and interdependence. The water defines and is altered by the obstacles – as in life, circumstances and environments are inextricably linked to the person's energy.

The river walls (*kawa no soku heki*) and floor (*kawa no zoko*) represent the environment, this could be the person's social environment (friends, family, work colleagues) or physical environment – the individual person indicates what is important to him/her. The rocks are those aspects of a person's life which are experienced as problematic and will vary in size, position and number. The drift wood represents personal attributes such as values, character traits, particular skills or material goods – those aspects of the self which can negatively or positively affect the person's life energy. Symbolically the rocks can block the river possibly severely impeding both the flow and the passage of driftwood; blockages suggest disharmony.

The model is also concerned with spaces (*sukima*) between all the elements in the river – as it is between these spaces that the river or life force continues to flow. The spaces provide the focus for occupational therapy because they suggest areas which the person values and considers as worthwhile. It is in these areas that the person continues to expend some energy. In more common occupational therapy terminology these could be interests or roles. And because the water flows in many different areas so occupational therapy is developed in many ways and on different levels, in close connection with the person and their context. Thus healing is not linear but is multi-faceted and one change in one area will affect another area. This model helps us to see this as a unified whole.

Justification for Kawa model

As culturally, both Karen and therapist were from England they interpreted and used the models in different ways from its original intention, and came to it with different values and beliefs. Nevertheless, the reasons for opting to use this model were:

- It has a theory base which shares commonality with self-in-relation theory and thus has some support from another theoretical frameworks found to be helpful for experiences of CSA (Holz 1994).
- It takes an egalitarian position and as such is very client-centred – the power and control lay with the Karen, and both Karen and therapist had freedom to interpret and adapt the model over time and according to changing needs.
- The model incorporates room for creative expression.

Basing reasoning on reading, Claire was guided by the document *Women's Mental Health: Into the Mainstream* (DoH 2002) which underlines the importance of working with and listening to women's subjective experiences.

Possible disadvantages

The Kawa model is a newly developed model therefore its clinical use in the UK has been limited. Some people may find its open and fluid structure difficult and the 'flowery' language and concepts may be culturally alien. In these circumstances another model would be more useful and accessible.

Claire's knowledge of Karen also helped to guide her choice of model as Karen could think symbolically (be able to attach meanings to objects) and had a strong interest in creative activities. Karen was reticent to talk but when the model was explained to Karen she appeared interested and after some hesitation responded positively to the metaphors of the river and rocks, and the model's inherent freedom of expression.

Task box 3

- Identify another occupational therapy model which could have been useful to Karen and the therapist.
- Outline your reasons.
- List three possible advantages of your choice and three possible disadvantages.

Implementation of the Kawa (river) model

In a quiet and private room in the day hospital, Karen, with Claire's guidance, drew out two cross-sections of Karen's river as a means of helping them both to find out Karen's perception of her life at this moment in time (Figures 5.2 and 5.3). This task proved to be therapeutic in itself and was also an important part of the initial assessment process. Figure 5.2 shows the obstructions to Karen's energy (family dynamics, unhelpful feelings, limited worthwhile activities and fears about going out) that served to block the assets which Karen had identified (kindness, sense of humour, IT skills). Because these had become obstructed she found that they were less accessible to her. Figure 5.3 shows the gaps between obstructions and assets which Karen labelled: feeling stronger; making friends; wanting to learn a new skill; cat owner. In the terms of the model as described by Iwama these spaces provide the impetus for occupational therapy.

This gave an overall picture of Karen's current needs as she saw them and in a form that was relevant to Karen and her creative nature. But to gain a more precise knowledge of Karen's needs, further assessment was necessary. Following discussion with Karen and the team, Claire decided to use a non-standardised approach to assessment as the clinical psychologist had used a range of standardised measures including Beck's Depression Inventory II (Beck 1961, revised 1996), Beck Hopelessness Scale (Beck 1987) and Mobility Inventory for Agorophobia (Chambless *et al.* 1985). Any changes in measurements were seen to be a reflection of the whole process rather than just a single intervention, and such information was shared with the whole team. Over a period of two weeks the assessments were carried out (see Table 5.2).

Task box 4

- Identify two other types of assessments which may have been useful to Karen.
- Outline your reasons.

Following the assessment Claire and Karen drew up a more detailed list of Karen's occupational strengths and needs (see Table 5.3). From this they negotiated an intervention plan, including short and long term aims, and steps required to meet these (see Table 5.4).

Issues for therapists

Literature is unanimous in its call for health workers to consider their own feelings and attitudes towards sexual abuse. Women who have experienced abuse are sensitive to the responses of others and therapists can inadvertently betray trust through lack of knowledge of dynamics associated with abuse (Foulder-Hughes 1998). It is therefore beholden upon us to take and if necessary seek opportunities to further our understanding of CSA and to consider our own feelings towards

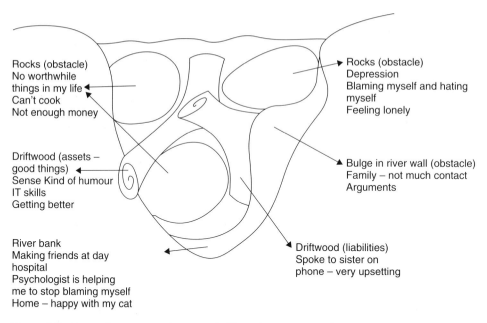

Rocks (obstacle)
No worthwhile
things in my life
Can't cook
Not enough money

Rocks (obstacle)
Depression
Blaming myself and hating
myself
Feeling lonely

Driftwood (assets –
good things)
Sense Kind of humour
IT skills
Getting better

Bulge in river wall (obstacle)
Family – not much contact
Arguments

River bank
Making friends at day
hospital
Psychologist is helping
me to stop blaming myself
Home – happy with my cat

Driftwood (liabilities)
Spoke to sister on
phone – very upsetting

Figure 5.2 Obstructions: preventing Karen's life and energy move forwards.

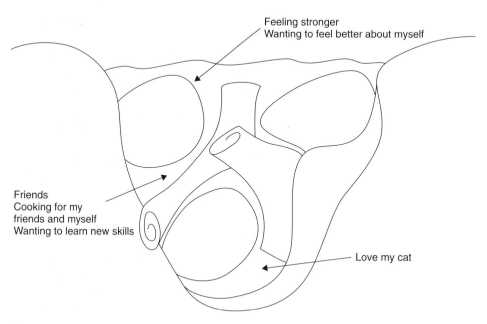

Feeling stronger
Wanting to feel better about myself

Friends
Cooking for my
friends and myself
Wanting to learn new skills

Love my cat

Figure 5.3 Spaces: potential for occupational therapy.

Table 5.2 Occupational therapy assessment process.

Assessment method	Reasoning	Outcome
Interest check list	Useful tool as a basis for establishing and discussing Karen's interests	Indicated creative activities as major interest – doing painting, writing poetry and visiting art galleries/shops Enjoys reality TV shows
Cooking assessment 1:1 in PDH kitchen, venue chosen as Karen had little equipment in her flat. Karen chose to cook spaghetti bolognaise, following discussion and looking at cookery books. Those with pictures and practical simple meals were most useful at this stage	Functional assessment which would enable Karen to have satisfaction of end product while also assessing her practical skills Emphasis on pleasurable activity rather than a test	Decided what to cook, with reassurance that it was within her capabilities Followed recipe with minimal prompts Issue appeared to be of confidence rather than limited skills Used sharp knife responsibly NB Karen lives at home therefore needed to be realistic regarding risk, important to help her to take positive risks while also monitoring her mood and adjusting activities accordingly
Shopping assessment Karen had had panic attacks at the supermarket – this was short walk from her flat but she had relied on small local shop for food Usually meant eating pot noodles or bacon sandwich This functional assessment was towards the end of the formal assessment period and followed visits to Karen's local shop	In vitro assessment of Karen's performance at the local supermarket. Karen had been having CBT for four weeks at this point and had developed strategies to help her deal with panic Important for her to face and move on from her fears in order for her to achieve her goals – Karen could see value in this	Anxious prior to leaving, (a shopping list had been prepared in advance to minimise anxiety) and on way to supermarket, used positive self-talk (I can cope with this, I am in control) and breathing exercises. Claire offering encouragement and minimal prompts Successfully completed task with two moments of panic when Karen could not find what she needed. Discussion followed to reinforce success and discuss what helped when feeling panicky

PDH, psychiatric day hospital; CBT, cognitive-behavioural therapy.

Table 5.3 Karen's occupational needs and strengths.

Needs	Strengths
More variety of productive activities and roles	Identifies positive qualities (kindness, good sense of humour)
Financial assessment	Recognises improvements made
Develop cookery skills and confidence	Identifies skills and areas she would like to develop
More support from family?	Using help provided, taking active part
Continue to externalise feelings – especially anger	Looking after her cat – a specific role and important source of comfort
Practise coping strategies especially when outside	

Table 5.4 Intervention plan and implementation.

Aims and objectives	Implementation
Short-term aim: To develop leisure interests outside PDH	Karen's strong interest in art was the focus of the first aim
(1) To continue attending weekly art group at PDH (1–6 weeks).	Open art group, twice weekly. Aim of group is to develop creative skills; gain confidence in materials and develop social interaction through art work. Group is planned and structured to maximise this, e.g. projects with a group focus
(2) By end of week 2 to visit Springfields Day Centre with OTA	Prior to discharge joined some of the groups at Springfield Day Centre. This was known to be a welcoming and encouraging place to go. In preparation at prearranged time Karen met with two of the staff and users, was shown around the centre and given information about the centre. Karen liked the place and agreed to attending art and IT groups
(3) By end of week 4 to walk to local shop to purchase some art materials to use at home	Although there was concern that art can be an isolating activity Karen had found painting a useful release and was a strong interest. Karen made list of materials and successfully bought what she needed
(4) By end of week 5 Karen to travel on bus to visit art gallery	This involved grading over a period of three weeks to help desensitise Karen to a short bus journey. As previously Karen recollected and used strategies to help her control any feelings of panic

Evidence: From their experience both Froehlich (1992) and Gillette (1996) support the use of creative activities with women who have experienced abuse and suggest many women find it useful for emotional expression. Creek (2003) and Sadlo (2004) both outline benefits of creative engagement

Table 5.4 *Continued*

Aims and objectives	Implementation
Short-term aim: To develop a productive role	Successful achievement of the first two objectives, gave Karen energy to research volunteering
(1) By end of week 3 to decide on type of voluntary work and to make enquiries	Decided to work for one of the animal welfare charity shops
(2) By end of week 4 to get telephone number and phone to find out more information	
(3) By end of week 5 to make specific arrangements for starting voluntary work (number of days, hours, where, type of work)	Made telephone call and arranged initially for two half days per week in the shop, mainly sorting and pricing items at first. Karen was satisfied with these arrangements and was pleased that the co-ordinator had shown interest in her IT skills

Evidence: Voluntary work is an increasingly accepted pathway into open employment or to provide meaningful occupation in its own right. Rebeiro and Allen (1998) outline a range of benefits to an individual with schizophrenia. For women who have been abused there are likely to be positive benefits to self-esteem, and self-identity as a volunteer worker

Aims and objectives	Implementation
Short-term aim: To develop cookery skills	Following on from the assessments, Karen wanted to cook a meal for two friends
(1) To plan and cook a meal for three with help from OTA at end of week 2	This involved deciding what to cook (within budget); shopping for ingredients and any equipment, cooking the meal in Karen's own kitchen; and helping Karen to prepare herself and flat for the occasion. The OT helped Karen to think through how she might approach the evening given that she had not seen her friends since the admission to hospital

Evidence: Limited specific research evidence for social meal cookery. But is more generally supported by client-centred practice; self-in-relation theory and Kawa (river) model, as this activity supports the value Karen places on her friendships and facilitates their connection

Aims and objectives	Implementation
Long-term aim: Employment and/or training course	Referral to specialist agency, support from mental health service if required

abuse through supervision networks and local professional support groups, if we are to be sensitive and effective occupational therapists with women who have survived childhood sexual abuse.

As with all mental health practice this sort of work can be emotionally draining. Listening to, believing, responding and checking one's own responses can be exhausting, especially where the stories are particularly distressing. This means good support and supervision networks are vital.

Evaluation, discharge and follow-up

Karen successfully achieved her occupational therapy aims with some minor alterations along the way and she developed skills and occupations to help her both now and in the future. By working together Lisa and Claire were able to help Karen make most of both parts of the intervention – reassessment using tools administered by Lisa reflected a positive change in Karen's mood.

   However Karen is not representative of all women who have survived CSA. She was at a point in her recovery when she could make most use of services and had positive life and personal resources to draw on. This will not be the same for everyone but meeting basic conditions of partnership, collaboration, flexibility and providing opportunities for Karen to exert control and creative expression meant occupational therapy played an important part in her recovery.

References

Abraham, V. (1998) Do occupational therapists feel equipped to deal with the adult legacy of childhood sexual abuse? *British Journal of Occupational Therapy.* **61**: 63–7.

Beck, A.T. (1961, revised 1996) *Beck Depression Inventory.* London: The Psychological Corporation.

Beck, A.T. (1987) *Beck Hopelessness Scale.* London: The Psychological Corporation.

Binder, R.L., McNiel, D.E. and Goldstone, R.L. (1996) Is adaptive coping for adult survivors of childhood sexual abuse? *Psychiatric Services.* **147**: 186–8.

Bohn, D. and Holz, K. (1996) Sequelae of abuse, health effects of child sexual abuse, domestic battering and rape. *Journal of Midwifery.* **41**: 442–56.

Chambless, D.L., Caputo, G.C., Jasin, S.E., Gracely, E.J. and Williams, C. (1985) The Mobility Inventory for Agoraphobia. *Behaviour Research and Therapy* **23**: 35–44.

COT (2005) *The Code of Ethics and Professional Conduct.* London: College of Occupational Therapists Ltd.

Coker, L. (1990) A therapeutic recovery model for the female adult incest survivor. Issues. *Mental Health Nursing.* **11**: 109–23.

Creedy, D., Nizette, D. and Henderson, K. (1998) A framework for practice with women survivors of childhood sexual abuse. *Australian and New Zealand Journal of Mental Health Practice.* **7**: 67–73.

Creek, J. (2003) Approaches to practice. In: Creek, J. (ed.) *Occupational Therapy and Mental Health,* 3rd edn. Edinburgh: Churchill Livingstone.

DoH (1999) *National Service Framework for Mental Health: Modern Standards and Service Models.* London: Department of Health.

DoH (2002) *Women's Mental Health: Into the Mainstream.* London: Department of Health.

Finkelhor, D. (1982) Sexual abuse. a sociological perspective. *Child Abuse and Neglect.* **6**: 95–102.

Finkelhor, D., Hotaling, G., Lewis, I. and Smith, C. (1990) Sexual abuse in a national survey of adult men and women: prevalence, characteristics and risk factors. *Child Abuse and Neglect.* **14**: 19–28.

Foulder-Hughes, L. (1998) The educational needs of occupational therapists who work with adult survivors of childhood sexual abuse. *British Journal of Occupational Therapy.* **61**: 68–74.

Froehlich, J. (1992) Occupational interventions with survivors of sexual abuse. *Occupational Therapy in Health Care.* **8**: 1–25.

Gillette, J. (1996) Child sexual abuse: working with survivors. *Australian and New Zealand Journal of Mental Health Nursing.* **5**: 69–76.

Gilligan, C. (1982) *In a Different Voice.* Cambridge: Harvard University Press.

Glaister, J.A. and Abel, E. (2001) Experiences of women healing from childhood sexual abuse. *Archives of Psychiatric Nursing* **XV**: 188–94.

Griffiths, R. (1998) Drug users who were abused as children. In: Bear, Z. (ed.) *Good Practice Guide in Counselling People Who Have Been Abused.* London: Jessica Kingsley Publishers.

Hall, J.M. and Kondora, L.L. (1997) Beyond 'true' and 'false' memories: remembering and recovery in the survival of childhood sexual abuse. *Advances in Nursing Science* **19**: 37–54.

Herman, J.L. (1992) *Trauma and Recovery.* New York: Basic Books.

Holz, K. (1994) A practical approach to clients who are survivors of childhood sexual abuse. *Journal of Nurse Midwifery.* **39**: 13–18.

Hulme, P.A. and Grove, S.K. (1994) Symptoms of female survivors of child sexual abuse. *Issues in Mental Health Nursing.* **15**: 519–32.

Iwama, M.K. (2005) The Kawa (river) model. Nature, life flow, and the power of culturally relevant occupational therapy. In: Kronenberg, F., Simo Algado, S. and Pollard, N. (eds) *Occupational Therapy Without Borders, Learning From the Spirit Of Survivors.* London: Elsevier Churchill Livingstone.

Krenken, J., van Stolk, B. (1990) Incest victims: inadequate help by professionals. *Child Abuse and Neglect.* **14**: 253–63.

Long, A. and Smyth, A. (1998) The role of mental health nursing in the prevention of child sexual abuse and the therapeutic care of survivors. *Journal of Psychiatric and Mental Health Nursing.* **5**: 129–36.

Meekums, B. (2000) Group therapy for women survivors of child sexual abuse. *Speaking the Unspeakable.* London: Jessica Kingsley Publishers.

Monahan, K. and Forgash, C. (2000) Enhancing the health care experiences of adult female survivors of childhood sexual abuse. *Women and Health* **30**: 27–41.

Miller, J.B. (1976) *Towards a New Psychology of Women.* Boston: Beacon Press.

NICE (2004) *Depression: Management of Depression in Primary and Secondary Care.* London: National Institute for Clinical Excellence.

Palmer, J.L., Coleman, L., Chaloner, D., Oppenheimer, R. and Smith, J. (1993) Childhood sexual experiences with adults: a comparison of reports by women psychiatric patients and general practice attenders. *British Journal of Psychiatry.* **163**: 499–504.

Rebeiro, K.L. and Allen, J. (1998) Voluntarism as occupation. *Canadian Journal of Occupational Therapy.*

Russell, D. (1986) *The Secret Trauma: Incest in the Lives of Girls and Women.* New York: Basic Books.

Sadlo, G. (2004) Creativity and occupation. In: Molineux, M. (ed.) *Occupation for Occupational Therapists.* Oxford: Blackwell.

Schachter, C.L., Rodomsky, N.A., Stalker, C.A. and Teram, E. (2004) Women survivors of child sexual abuse. How can health professionals promote healing? *Canadian Family Physician.* **50**: 405–12.

Sheldon, H. (1998) Childhood sexual abuse in adult female psychotherapy referrals. Incidence and implications for treatment. *British Journal of Psychiatry.* **152**: 107–11.

Williams, J. (2005) Women's mental health, taking inequality into account. In: Tew, J. (ed.) *Social Perspectives in Mental Health.* London: Jessica Kingsley Publishers.

Wolf, R. (1998) Becoming real: The story of a long journey through psychiatry, counselling and psychotherapy. In: Bear, Z. (ed.) *Good Practice Guide in Counselling People Who Have Been Abused.* London: Jessica Kingsley Publishers.

Further reading

Holz, K. (1994) A practical approach to clients who are survivors of childhood sexual abuse. *Journal of Nurse Midwifery.* **39**: 13–18.
This paper gives a clear and readable account of possible issues for women who have been subjected to sexual abuse, with specific consideration for pregnancy and child birth. Not directly relevant to occupational therapy practice but could be useful basis for collaborating with nursing colleagues and deepening knowledge of professional roles.

Health Canada (2001) *Handbook on Sensitive Practice for Health Professionals: Lessons from Women Survivors of Childhood Sexual Abuse.* Available at: www.phac-aspc.gc.ca/ncfv-cnivf/familyviolence/pdfs/handbook_e.pdf.
An excellent practical guide to working with survivors of CSA. Downloadable and comprehensive, it gives easy to follow guidance on a range of issues, interspersed with comments from women who have been abused and have used health care services.

Itzen, C. (2006) *Tackling the Health and Mental Health Effects of Domestic and Sexual Violence and Abuse.* London: Department of Health.
As its title suggests, this document aims to equip services and professionals to identify and respond to the needs of people affected by violence and abuse, regardless of age, diagnosis, gender or whether victim or abuser.

6: Personality disorder: occupational therapy inclusion

Jane Cronin-Davis

Occupational therapy, while relatively new to forensic mental health is a well-established and recognised profession. Forensic mental health services have, according to Wix and Humphreys (2005, p. xi), been 'developing apace over the last decade or more'. Since the 1990s there has been an increasing demand for occupational therapists to work with offenders with mental disorders or patients detained in secure hospital settings (Crawford 2003) and the specific contribution of the profession has been recognised (Chacksfield 1997, Flood 1997, Baker and McKay 2001, Humphreys 2005). The Reed Report (Department of Health (DoH) and Home Office 1992) made specific recommendations for the care and services required for offenders with mental disorders, with a strong emphasis on rehabilitation and independence. This report suggested that high-quality care should be provided with due attention to individual needs; wherever possible individuals should be cared for in the community; security levels should be proportionate to the identified risk of an individual; and finally individuals should be cared for as close as possible to their own home and family.

The term 'forensic' can be defined as relating to courts of law (*Oxford Dictionary* 2005) and therefore related to criminal or offending behaviour. However, there is considerable debate about what actually constitutes forensic care. Forensic mental health is considered to be the specialist clinical area responsible for patients with mental health problems who have had or will have contact with the legal system, an uneasy alliance at times. Forensic environments include high, medium and low secure hospitals or units and more recently, forensic community teams (see Wix and Humphreys (2005) for a very good overview of the historical development of forensic services in the UK). The ultimate goal of forensic services is usually for the individual patient to re-integrate back into the community with a comprehensive care and treatment programme which addresses ongoing needs and risk management (Cronin-Davis *et al.* 2004). A helpful definition provided by Woods (2002) suggests that forensic care needs to create a safe and therapeutic environment, one that considers risk and anger management, avoids labelling and provided offence-related interventions.

It has been suggested that the forensic population typically consists of white, single men from lower socioeconomic groups who have generally not worked prior to admission (Thompson *et al.* 1997). For many patients in high, medium or low secure hospitals, their occupational abilities, choices and opportunities have been eroded due to the effects of often long-term institutionalisation. Some patients may have had limited opportunities to develop a sense of themselves as competent occupational beings due to the impact of the contexts in which they grew up and lived (Cronin-Davis *et al.* 2004).

The role of occupational therapists in forensic settings has been well defined by Couldrick and Aldred (2003) as the treatment of people with mental health problems who offend; they recognise that by helping people to engage in occupations which give their lives meaning and value this may mitigate against offending and antisocial behaviour. Humphreys (2005) states that forensic occupational therapists have, in some cases, more day-to-day contact with patients than any other professional. Blackburn (1996) asserts that in forensic settings it is important to remember that rehabilitation should not be limited to teaching patients skills for domestic tasks and occupational therapists need to be cognisant of this when planning occupational therapy programmes. Cronin-Davis *et al.* (2004) emphasise that occupational therapists must acknowledge the impact of a patient's forensic pathology; and they must ensure occupational therapy interventions not only recognise the risks involved and formulate treatment, but that they are also proactive in addressing how patients' criminal occupations impact on their life style and well-being. This is the unique contribution of occupational therapy within this clinical speciality.

The purpose of this chapter is to introduce you to Sally and describe her occupational therapy intervention with a young man called Joe, who had been admitted to a specialist forensic medium secure unit for men diagnosed with a personality disorder. The chapter will explore how Sally chose to provide occupational therapy intervention. It will discuss some of the issues she faced trying to adhere to her core occupational therapy principles and philosophy and balancing client-centred practice in a restrictive environment which is often more focused on the management of risk. Despite the call for client centredness in occupational therapy literature, the term patient will be used throughout this chapter as this indicates Joe's legal status as a patient detained under the Mental Health Act 1983.

Sally's new post – forensic occupational therapy

Sally had been qualified for approximately 18 months; her first post was in acute mental health on an admission ward and the second in a community mental health team. She had always been interested and had more of a leaning towards mental health ever since she was a student. Sally had specifically chosen to apply for a job in forensic mental health because she had heard from colleagues that it was both an interesting and a challenging clinical area with a strong focus on multi-disciplinary working. She was aware that at times it would not be an easy environment. However, within the occupational therapy team, she would have a number of more senior experienced occupational therapists who could offer her guidance and support when she needed it. The team comprised of a head of service, four senior and two junior occupational therapists, with technical instructors for sports and leisure, horticulture, art, pottery and work skills. To complement the team, there were administration staff and education and information technology tutors.

Before she was able to start working on the ward and with the patients, Sally participated in the unit's induction programme. This covered such topics such as the management of violence and aggression (recognition and de-escalation skills), breakaway techniques (skills for escaping a situation quickly and efficiently without the use of undue force), control and restraint (physical skills for the management of violence), Mental Health Act and relevant legislation, risk assessment and management, and effective therapeutic relationships (boundary setting, supervision, personal disclosure and safety), basic life support, and legal and child protection issues.

Reflection

How else do you think Sally could prepare herself for working in a forensic setting?

What do you think are some of the important issues Sally will need to consider in relation to her clinical practice?

What do you think some of the tensions might be with regards to the holistic nature of occupational therapy practice and the restrictions of a secure hospital setting?

The setting

The unit took account of a range of guidelines which have been issued relevant to forensic and mental health practice. Most pertinent was *Personality Disorder: No Longer a Diagnosis of Exclusion* (National Institute of Mental Health in England (NIMHE) 2003a), a policy implementation guide for developing services for people with the personality disorder diagnosis. It sets out to: emphasise the unique needs of people with a personality disorder diagnosis who experience significant distress and a need to access appropriate clinical care and management; ensure offenders with a personality disorder diagnosis receive care from relevant forensic services which address both their clinical needs and offending behaviour; and establish the education and training necessary to enable practitioners with the skills needed in assessment and management.

This was a useful document for Sally to read as it gave many suggestions about possible places to visit, helpful and unhelpful characteristics of services, what service users feel they need, and what treatments are considered helpful. There are useful appendices to this document and the recommendations are supported by relevant literature and research. The guideline makes it clear that forensic services should focus on treatment and management of social functioning, mental health issues, offending behaviour and risk. It is also highlighted some of the legal issues which Sally needed to be aware of.

Due to the nature of the disorder, there was also the potential for some patients to be disturbed, challenging or violent. Key guidance for the short-term management of violent/disturbed behaviour has been published by the National Institute for Health and Clinical Excellence (NICE 2005) to assist practitioners. Key priorities for implementation included training, prediction, working with service users, rapid tranquillisation, physical interventions and seclusion. Particular reference is given to the importance of the environment and use of therapeutic activities (Cronin-Davis 2005). Sally made a note of these issues realising that this would be an important facet of her work on the psychiatric day unit (PDU).

The PDU worked on the premise of a 'structured therapeutic day'. All patients were expected to get up by 8.00 am and attend a morning community meeting where they planned their day and were informed of visitors to the ward, events on the ward or in the hospital. There were therapeutic groups facilitated on the ward by occupational therapy and nursing staff. Trips when relevant were discussed at the morning meeting. The daily therapeutic programme ended by 5.00 pm and patients were expected to use their free time in the evenings on their own projects, therapy tasks or spending time winding down.

Reflection

- What other official documents or guidelines would it be useful for Sally to read?
- What are some of the legal implications Sally would need to consider?
- How would you start thinking about which occupational therapy treatment interventions would be most suitable?

The multi-disciplinary team

The occupational therapy team was well established as members of a multi-disciplinary clinical team and were all based on specific wards. The ward-based team consisted of a consultant forensic psychiatrist, a forensic psychologist, a pharmacist, a senior social worker, a ward manager, nursing staff and domestic staff, and an occupational therapist (Sally). The multi-disciplinary team was fairly new as there had been a number of staff changes and skill mix, therefore the team members were in the process of learning about the skills and expertise individual team members could bring to the team. Humphreys (2005) discusses the need for unique professional expertise and experience in the field of forensic mental health; he acknowledges that there may be areas of role overlap and considers this useful if the team can be open and frank with honest communication. Humphreys believes that this can aid the effective sharing of work and responsibility, teamworking, decision-making, with a sense of inclusion and empowerment. To try to achieve this the team met weekly to discuss clinical governance and business issues; in addition they met as a clinical team to discuss and review patients' clinical pathways and high on the clinical agenda were discussions about individual patients' risk assessment and risk management, and the Care Programme Approach (DoH 1990).

The patients were also considered to be part of the team in terms of negotiating and planning their own care, and decision-making regarding certain operational aspects of the ward. There was a ward representative who met with other ward representatives on a monthly basis and discussed issues with the occupational therapy team. This group was responsible for organising weekend and evening social activities for the patients.

There was also a strong patient advocacy group in the hospital.

Reflection

It might be useful for you to read around the subject of advocacy and consider why it is important to have advocacy groups for patients in forensic settings.

Personality disorder – understanding the diagnosis and implications for occupational therapy

Personality disorder: for some a complex, perplexing and stigmatising diagnosis. However, more positively, it can be considered a sign-post which can help direct the appropriate assessment and intervention strategies. Historically, people with this diagnosis were deemed untreatable by professionals or agencies involved in their care, or too difficult to treat as their demands on professionals can seem overwhelming. They were often considered unmotivated to change and accept responsibility for themselves. Often, little acknowledgement is given to the turmoil, distress and psychological pain which may be experienced by those who attract this seemingly pejorative label (Cronin-Davis 2004). Personality disorders are seemingly common conditions, the estimates for prevalence vary from 10% to 13% in the adult population; in mental health hospitals the figures rise to 36–67% (NIMHE 2003b). Singleton and colleagues (1998) suggest the figure for adult prisoners is estimated at 50–78% and two-thirds of offenders with mental disorders are believed to have more than one personality disorder diagnosis (Blackburn *et al.* 2003).

When Sally read the NIMHE (2003a) document *Personality Disorder: No Longer a Diagnosis of Exclusion* she noted the inference it made – that many people with personality disorder can negotiate the tasks of daily living, however, some suffer a great deal of distress and can place a heavy burden on family, friends and carers. But what are the characteristics of the diagnosis? Sally felt she needed to know more. The definition given by the *International Classification of Mental and Behavioural Disorders* 10th revision (ICD-10) (World Health Organization (WHO) 1993) is as follows:

> '*A severe disturbance in the characterological condition and behavioural tendencies of the individual, usually involving several areas of the personality, and nearly always associated with considerable personal and social disruption.*'

The *American Diagnostic and Statistical Manual of Mental Disorders* (DSM-IV) (American Psychiatric Association (APA) 1994), however, offers a more extensive diagnosis and labelled as Axis II disorders:

> 'an enduring pattern of inner experience and behaviour that deviates markedly from the expectations of the individual's culture, is pervasive and inflexible, has an onset in adolescence or early adulthood, is stable over time, and leads to distress or impairment.'

From the author's own experience of working with clients with a personality disorder diagnosis, it is true to note that many people diagnosed with personality disorder will have experienced significant trauma in their early years with associated attachment difficulties. The different types of personality disorder are detailed in Table 6.1. Some of the implications for occupational therapy practice are identified by Bonder (2004) and Stein and Cutler (2002). Bonder suggests that patients with a personality disorder can be helped by group programmes which focus on co-operation and social skills training. Realistic self-appraisal and self-awareness may be difficult and occupations which focus on developing self-esteem and being appreciated by others should be facilitated. Table 6.1 gives an overview of the commonest types of personality disorder and possible implications for occupational therapy practice. In the DSM-IV system the personality disorder diagnoses are often referred to as cluster A, B or C.

Although Table 6.1 outlines the main features and possible implications for occupational therapy practice, Sally was acutely aware that she should not stereotype patients according to their diagnosis or diagnoses, as often patients in forensic mental health may have more than one personality disorder diagnosis or traits. One of the most important features to be acknowledged is the many challenges associated with working with patients diagnosed with a personality disorder. For example, it has been suggested that they are likely to 'compromise therapeutic relationships' (UKCC 1999). People with personality disorder can suffer distressing and stigmatising attitudes from staff involved in their care, when all they request is understanding and patience (Thoughts of service users 2003). The challenges and concerns associated with working with people are well documented (Fraser and Gallop 1993, Duff *et al.* 2003, Warren *et al.* 2003, Murphy and McVey 2003). However, positive and exciting opportunities exist for developing clinical practice and expertise with this very deserving group of patients. Therapeutic endeavour and optimism are key qualities of those involved in the care and treatment of people with personality disorder, and Sally was keen to focus on this.

Reflection

There are a number of competing and emerging theories as to the exact origin and development of personality disorder but these are beyond the remit of this chapter. The reader may find helpful the list of further reading at the end of the chapter.

What are some of the other theories Sally might consider to assist her understanding of the diagnosis and the implications for occupational therapy practice?

Table 6.1 Classification of personality disorders and implications for occupational therapy practice.

ICD-10 diagnosis	DSM-IV diagnosis	Main features	Implications for occupational therapy practice (source: Bonder 2004, Stein and Cutler 2002)
Cluster A			
Paranoid personality disorder	Paranoid personality disorder	Excessively sensitive and can misinterpret the actions of others	Inter-personal difficulties cause problems in work and social settings. Inaccurate processing of social cues Few leisure interests
Schizoid personality disorder	Schizoid personality disorder	Emotionally cold and withdrawn Introspective Restricted range of emotions and expressions	Impaired social relationships may prefer occupations involving mechanical, computer or mathematical tasks
No equivalent	Schizotypal personality disorder	Odd beliefs and thinking Difficulties relating to people; and often unusual behaviour	Social functioning is poor Vocational functioning is impaired if social skills are necessary to employment
Cluster B			
Dissocial personality disorder	Anti-social personality disorder	Aggressive, unstable, impulsivity, lying and manipulation Lack of concern and empathy for others Difficulties in relationships Tendency for criminal behaviour	Work and social functioning impaired Impaired social relationships due to lack of concern for others Finances may be a problem; stealing may be one way used to compensate
Emotional unstable personality disorder (impulsive, borderline)	Borderline personality disorder	Difficulties managing anger, marked feelings of emptiness, pervasive instability of mood, emotional outbursts and suicidal ideation. Fear of abandonment Depersonalisation	Difficulties with inter-personal relationships and self-image, often present with self-harming behaviour Vocational and social functioning are often impaired Difficulties setting and following goals. High risk of suicide

Table 6.1 *Continued*

ICD-10 diagnosis	DSM-IV diagnosis	Main features	Implications for occupational therapy practice (source: Bonder 2004, Stein and Cutler 2002)
Histrionic personality disorder	Histrionic personality disorder	Egocentricity, attention-seeking, dramatic, crave excitement and persistent manipulative behaviour Explosive personality reactions	Social functioning, friendships may be superficial and focus on the individual Can function at work but are often a problem to supervisors and co-workers
No equivalent	Narcissistic personality disorder	Grandiosity, self-importance, with a strong desire for admiration from others Lacks empathy towards others	Poor inter-personal relationships, brief and often contentious Rarely develop insight into their behaviour as there is tendency to blame others for their problems Often have problems in work situations – performance may be good as the individual strives for success; however it may also be poor due to the perceived expectations of others, which is resented
Cluster C Anankastic personality disorder	Obsessive compulsive personality disorder	Indecisive, doubting excessive caution Pre-occupied with orderliness and perfectionism	Pre-occupations can interfere with the completion of tasks Occupational balance impaired Never feel as if they have achieved or done well enough Social and vocational impairments Individuals can be aware of their behaviour leading to depression
Anxious (avoidant) personality disorder	Avoidant personality disorder	Persistent social avoidance and discomfort, timid, hypersensitive to rejection	Work and self-care often unaffected, but difficulties forming relationships, tendency to be a loner
Dependent personality disorder	Dependent personality disorder	Avoid relationships Subordinates to the needs of others Excessive dependence on others and fails to take responsibility for self	Difficulties making decisions and look to others for guidance Find it difficult to initiate occupations and to be objective about themselves

To prepare herself for her new post, Sally carried out research and background reading. She found texts such as *Forensic Occupational Therapy* (Couldrick and Aldred 2003) with a chapter by Couldrick (2003) helpful. Couldrick suggests that skill deficits for people with personality disorder tend to be in the cognitive, and intra- and inter-personal skills. Sally was also keen to establish the precise evidence base for occupational therapy intervention for people with personality disorders. Sally located articles relating to occupational therapy and personality disorder dating from 1955 to 2004. The first was by Dr Noyes (1955). He suggested that occupational therapists must focus on socialisation, developing patients abilities and 'stimulating interest in new activities'. In addition he suggested that therapists must show concern, personal interest and understanding, a sentiment strongly echoed in contemporary literature. These articles were of interest to read and somewhat useful in considering the use of activities and the Model of Human Occupation. Cara (1992) gave an overview of the programme used with people diagnosed with narcissistic personality disorder and an explanation of possible interpersonal responses to patients. This was, however, an anecdotal description. So the information thus far had not been robust research evidence. However, Sally then found a paper by Lindstedt and colleagues (2004) who report on a study carried out in Sweden with mentally disordered offenders (n = 161), examining their abilities in occupational performance and social participation. The research demonstrated that mentally disordered offenders, including those with a personality disorder diagnosis, had a limited awareness of their own abilities; they also reported that personality disordered patients in the study had longstanding 'disablements that caused major difficulties in everyday life in the last two to three years'. They concluded that their results suggest mentally disordered offenders need support to live in the community.

The limited amount of relevant published research-based literature was a dilemma for Sally in her quest to be an evidence-based practitioner: she found little to help her specifically with her work in a forensic unit with patients with personality disorder. She discussed this with colleagues and, although there is strong emphasis on evidence-based practice in today's clinical arena, Sally recognised that occupational therapy could still be an effective clinical intervention for patients with personality disorder. She was reminded and reassured by the writings of Taylor (2000) who states that:

> *'external evidence is just one strand of the process and must be blended with clinical judgement and patient preference.'*

Theory and practice

Sally was well aware of the occupational therapy team's strong focus on occupational science as a foundation for understanding humans as occupational beings. She knew that the team was rooted in the belief that occupation and the human need to engage in occupation could be one key to a patient's improvement. Occupational science can provide a framework to understand the complexities of patients in forensic settings (Cronin-Davis *et al.* 2004, pp. 170–1). These authors suggest that the unique challenge for occupational therapists is to be cognisant of the risks posed by forensic patients while still facilitating occupational engagement in a creative and resourceful way relevant to the identified risks. In brief, the elements represented in Figure 6.1 can be defined as follows and will be used to outline Joe's occupational dysfunction later.

- *Homo occupacio.* A self-organising system which can respond to environmental challenges by using occupation and thereby creating an adaptive response. Adaptive and successful self-organisations develop skills which can be used in new or previously not encountered situations (Yerxa 2000).
- *Performance deficits* impact on an individual's ability at the occupational performance component level, for example sensorimotor, cognitive or psychosocial (Cronin-Davis *et al.* 2004).
- *Occupational disruption* is considered to be the transient or lasting inability to engage in occupations as a result of life events, acute illness, injury or environmental changes (Whiteford 1997).
- *Occupational deprivation* can be defined as the deprivation of occupational choices which are beyond the control of an individual (Wilcock 1998) and occurs over an extended period of time (Whiteford 1997).

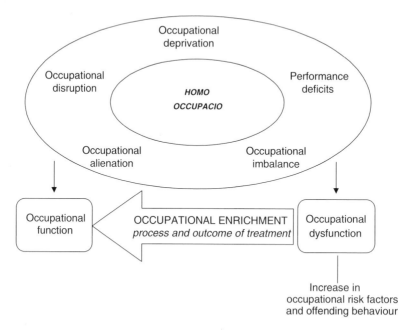

Figure 6.1 Conceptualising the occupational therapy process and occupational risk factors in forensic psychiatry. (Developed from the original work by Stockton Hall Hospital Occupational Therapy Service.) Reproduced from Molineux, M. (ed.) (2004) *Occupation for Occupational Therapists*, with permission from Blackwell Publishing.

Occupational alienation is thought to be a subjective experience where an individual may feel powerlessness, frustration, isolation, loss of control and estranged from society (Wilcock 1998).

Occupational imbalance. A loss of balance in those occupations which would normally be health-giving to an individual; and as Wilcock (1998) suggests a balance between physical, mental and social occupations, chosen or obligatory, or doing and being.

Occupational enrichment. This can be achieved by providing opportunities for patients to engage in a range of occupations either alone or within groups. It may also involve addressing wider systemic issues within forensic services or institutions, such as policies on access to the community, employment programmes and family contact opportunities. The ultimate aim of occupational therapy is to enable patients to experience occupational enrichment and thus achieve occupational functioning. It can however be hugely challenging within secure environments, therefore the skills of occupational therapists at devising treatment programmes with, and for, their clients require a more creative and versatile skill base (Cronin-Davis *et al.* 2004).

Although these factors may at times be prevalent for many individuals, they are still able to lead occupationally fulfilling lives, so what is it about those who come into contact with mental health services which make these more of a problem? Due to the nature and restrictions of the forensic environment, this can also compound occupational risk factors and further impact on an individual's occupational functioning and well-being (Cronin-Davis *et al.* 2004).

Joe – the patient

Joe had been transferred to the PDU from prison where he was serving a sentence for the attempted murder of his girlfriend. He was transferred under section 47/49 of the Mental Health Act 1983. This meant that Joe was a convicted prisoner and movement outside the secure hospital environment required permission from the Home Office.

Joe was 25 years old and had been in prison for three years. He had been referred for inpatient assessment and treatment of his mental health problems following medical diagnosis by the prison's visiting psychiatrist. Joe had been receiving some input from the prison in-reach mental health team who had tried to assess Joe. He found it difficult to engage with the team as he did not like the stigma of being associated with mental health professionals while in prison. However, it was felt that he needed a more comprehensive assessment and treatment package as the prison psychiatrist had diagnosed Joe with borderline personality disorder with anti-social traits. He was also suffering from social anxiety and had features of depression: low mood, poor sleep and diet, and a lack of interest in occupations. He had been isolating himself, was being verbally and sometimes physically aggressive to prison staff, and had been self-harming by burning himself with cigarettes, swallowing batteries and lacerating his arms. Sally wanted to try to understand some of the possible implications of Joe's diagnoses and had read around the subject.

In an attempt to make sense of Joe's background history and story by talking to him and reading background information from psychiatric and multidisciplinary pre-admission assessment reports, Sally also used her knowledge of individuals as occupational beings. Occupational science provides a framework which enables the occupational therapist to understand the complexities of patients in a forensic setting. It acknowledges the wider issues and external influences of a patient's circumstances and psychopathology, and provides a vehicle for the comprehensive exploration of risk factors (Cronin-Davis *et al.* 2004). Sally used the occupational risk factors identified earlier in this chapter to conceptualise aspects of Joe's case and his specific occupational needs.

Occupational deprivation

Joe was born to parents who were unable to care for him due to their own mental health and substance misuse problems. He was fostered from the age of nine months and spent many of his early years in a number of foster homes. He never knew his parents or his two older siblings who were also taken into care. At the age of 12, Joe was placed in a secure children's home as foster parents were finding it difficult to deal with his increasingly unruly and aggressive behaviour. He describes feeling unloved and unwanted. Due to the number of placements and his difficulty settling into schools, Joe found school very difficult and left with no educational achievements. When he was 16, Joe ran away from his final placement and lived on the streets in London. He made a living by stealing, begging and occasionally shop-lifting to order. He had no possessions, no stable social network and used illicit substances, mainly cocaine. Joe had never held a conventional job.

As a prisoner Joe was deprived of making any occupational choices for himself due to the nature of the prison environment. He lacked company and spent many hours locked up in his prison cell either watching television or listening to music on a small radio. Due to his aggressive behaviour, he often spent long periods in segregation. Now that he was in hospital, Sally was keen to try to engage Joe in occupations and therapeutic activities he might find stimulating and useful, however, she knew that she had to be careful not to impose this on him.

Occupational alienation

As a child, Joe always felt different from other children, due to the fact that his parents had abandoned him and he lived with numerous foster carers. He had no significant family attachments and was unaware of the whereabouts of his older brothers. Joe had experienced bullying as a child, with people referring to him as that 'dirty kid with no parents'. He had no significant relationships except for his girlfriend, Jess; they had met while they were both living rough in a large city. Jess was younger than Joe and relied on him to obtain drugs and alcohol. Theirs was a volatile and abusive relationship, with frequent arguments and violence towards one another. After a night of particularly heavy drinking and using crack cocaine, Joe stabbed Jess with a knife he carried with him for his own protection. This caused severe wounds to her chest and abdomen that necessitated surgery and a long stay in hospital.

While in prison, Joe was considered susceptible to bullying from other prisoners and kept on special units for vulnerable prisoners. However, due to his own frequently aggressive or hostile behaviour, he often spent time in the segregation units and was ostracised by both prison staff and the other prisoners. He was not allowed to work in the prison, although he did attend education from time to time. Joe did not have any friends or social visitors while in prison. He lacked a sense of autonomy and real self-identity. Joe also felt that others could look at him and detect what crime he had committed. Now, despite being in hospital with other patients with similar problems and background to himself, Joe still felt very different and could not identify with other patients.

Occupational imbalance

Due to his poor upbringing, Joe had experienced few occupational choices and his life style on the streets had been focused on surviving from day to day. He had to beg and steal to fund his drug habit.

In prison, Joe spent most of his days lying in his room. He would eat meals at allocated times and have a shower when he could. Apart from this his life focused on watching television, listening to music and reading. Because of his aggressive and disruptive behaviour Joe did not participate in social activities, 'association'. He had few friends and was not a popular prisoner and therefore left very much to his own devises in his prison cell.

In hospital, initially Joe found it very difficult to participate in the ward routine due his poor occupational balance. He was unable to decide what he would and would not participate in, he wanted to spend his time in his room as this is what he had been used to in the prison system.

Occupational disruption

His frequent placements as a child and subsequent life living on the streets meant that Joe was in a constant state of occupational disruption. He barely had time to settle in to a placement before he was moved, usually due to his behaviour. In prison, he was often moved from one prison to another again due to his perceived difficult behaviour and the prison staff felt it was difficult to manage him.

A 'blanket referral' system operated on the PDU, Sally was expected to carry out an occupational therapy assessment for all patients newly admitted to the ward. An occupational therapy report would contribute to the initial overall multi-disciplinary assessment of Joe; the quality standard for the Unit was set at three months for this initial assessment. The Unit also used its own locally developed risk assessment measure, to which Sally was expected to contribute.

Reflection

Before reading the next section, take some time to consider the occupational therapy process (see Duncan 2006, Chapter 4).

Also take some time to reflect on those occupational therapy models and frameworks for practice that you might use when working with patients such as Joe.

In her previous posts, Sally had used the Occupational Performance Process Model (Stanton *et al.* 2002) to facilitate occupational therapy practice with patients. Several key features of this generic process model can be used with all patients in a diversity of settings. It is applicable to the forensic setting as it is action orientated; there is a theory–practice link; it helps to differentiate occupational therapy from other disciplines; and finally this model acknowledges the expertise of both the patient and therapist and leads to client outcomes. By using the seven-stage process, Sally was able to work systematically in partnership with Joe, with a strong emphasis on client-centred practice. The seven stages will now be described to show how they were used in the occupational therapy intervention programme with Joe.

Stage one – name, validate and prioritise occupational performance

To assess Joe and consider areas for occupational therapy intervention, Sally began meeting with him within the first two days of admission. These took the form of informal 'get to know you' sessions before a more formal assessment process could start. Sally was aware that many patients in Joe's position have issues relating to trust and engagement with staff, and it was important to establish a professional and therapeutic relationship. Patients with personality disorder have reported experiencing unhelpful attitudes from staff, and being treated in a belittling or patronising manner; what they need is staff who can handle therapeutic relationships with people who may be vulnerable, dangerous and abusive, and staff who are truthful, respectful, interested and accepting (Thoughts of service users 2003).

Sally was aware from her knowledge about personality disorder characteristics and his history that it would be more likely that Joe would have problems relating to people, engaging in occupations, and intrapersonal skills. Sally needed to validate this with Joe and get his perception of his difficulties; she also needed to be aware of his risks.

Multi-disciplinary risk assessment is a key and vital component of mental health practice in the current mental health political and clinical climate. This has largely been driven by the need to protect the public. Both actuarial and clinical risk assessments are used in forensic mental health. Prior to his admission to the PDU, Joe's risk assessment had been carried out using the HCR-20 (Webster *et al.* 1997) and VRAG (Quinsey *et al.* 1998) and the PCL-R (Hare 1991) to assess his risk of violence. These are all examples of actuarial measures, i.e. measures and their data which refer to instruments or statistics based on what is known about violent behaviour (Jones and Plowman 2005). This is a rapidly developing science and continually new and more detailed assessments are being published. Practitioners are encouraged to keep abreast of the current developments, research and formulation criteria.

Reflection

Consider conducting a literature search regarding risk assessment in the area of forensic mental health. How many research tools have been validated for use in forensic mental health?

How does the process of risk assessment fit in with occupational therapy practice?

In terms of the process of a clinical risk assessment, Jones and Plowman (2005) state that this must be grounded in a full and detailed history of the individual. They suggest the following baseline information is necessary and can be obtained by the multi-disciplinary team: family background; educational history; occupational history; relationship history; psychiatric history; substance abuse history; and forensic history. Risk assessment itself is an ongoing, dynamic process and should not just be limited to the propensity for violence. Self-harm, suicide and suicidal ideation, neglect, substance misuse, sexual aggression/behaviour, arson, escape, absconding and hostage-taking are additional behaviours which need to be considered. Multi-disciplinary teams need to establish clear policies and guidelines regarding methods of assessment, completion, review and risk management plans. Sally was acutely aware of how important risk assessment was on the PDU and with practice began to develop confidence in helping to compile risk assessments and management plans. It was particularly pertinent for those patients who had sessions in high-risk areas, such as kitchens and workshops.

Joe's initial risk assessment identified that he could become violent and verbally aggressive in certain situations; he had the propensity to seriously self-harm if he was feeling out of control or unable to cope. Joe had expressed suicidal ideation in the past and he had tried to hang himself on one occasion (two years ago with his shoe laces while in prison). He had a long history of substance misuse. He had no documented history of sexual aggression, hostage-taking, or attempts to escape/abscond.

The team did not rely solely on self-report from Joe, and extensive efforts were made by relevant staff to gather as much background information and reports as were available so that the team could make informed decisions. Jones and Plowman

(2005) believe that multi-disciplinary risk assessment can be improved through effective team work, enabling responsibilities, tasks and information expertise to be shared. In addition, they suggest that support within the team means that no one individual team member is left to complete the difficult and time-consuming risk assessment process alone.

Stage two – select theoretical approaches

Although Sally had used the discipline of occupational science to understand Joe, the occupational therapy team used the Model of Human Occupation to facilitate practice (see Kielhofner 2002 for a detailed approach to the model). Anecdotally, it is well known within forensic occupational therapy as a useful model to help identify component areas of dysfunctional performance, and it focuses on the impact of the environment (see Duncan 2003, Forsyth and Kielhofner 2005).

Stage three – identify occupational performance components and environmental conditions

Sally used a variety of methods to gather information both from Joe and from the numerous reports which had been compiled (pre-admission, prison psychologist, prison healthcare wing documentation). As well as understanding Joe as an occupational being in his own right by using occupational science, Sally wanted to assess his occupational performance at a component level if necessary. To do this she carried out both an occupation-based assessment (Hocking 2001) and used a variety of assessments associated with the Model of Human Occupation (Kielhofner 2002): Occupational Performance History Interview – Version 2 (Kielhofner et al. 1998); Assessment of Communication and Interactions Skills (Forsyth et al. 1998); Occupational Therapy Task Observation Scale (Margolis 1996); Occupational Self Assessment (Baron et al. 1999). Sally used her clinical observation skills to assess Joe while he was on the main ward area, she asked him to attend the groups organised for patients on the ward and engaged him in individual sessions.

She discussed his participation and performance, and his non-participation in the ward-based groups facilitated by the activity organiser. Over a period of a few weeks, Sally began to build up a picture of Joe and used her clinical reasoning skills to understand the nature and possible origin of his performance difficulties. It was important that she shared her assessment findings with Joe for a number of reasons: to validate her findings and to establish whether her assessment concurred with Joe's perception of his difficulties. In addition to her information gathering, individual members of the clinical team discussed their assessment findings at the weekly clinical team meetings. At these meetings particular reference was paid to Joe's risk assessment and management.

It was obvious that Joe had many difficulties in relation to his self-esteem, self-identity, and occupational engagement. He found it difficult to 'label' his emotions. Joe also had major problems identifying occupations which he would find interesting and beneficial. Joe agreed with Sally that he was socially anxious and that this prevented him from engaging in therapeutic activities. His personality difficulties also made it hard for him to accept praise and encouragement. Joe would try to push people away by being verbally aggressive before they could get close to him. The long-standing issues meant that he had difficulties trusting therapists and staff.

Due to his potential risks of self-harm and aggressive/disturbed behaviour, Sally had to carefully consider the environments in which therapy could take place. The occupational therapy team and multi-disciplinary team operated with a positive risk-taking culture provided a patient's risks could be identified and managed safely, this was in keeping with the concept of occupational enrichment.

Stage four – identify strengths and resources (client's strengths and external resources)

Despite being relatively new to the clinical area of personality disorder, Sally was a keen and enthusiastic therapist and embraced the notion of client-centred practice. She wanted to provide Joe with appropriate occupational experiences, and thus she was a resource for Joe. She was willing to look for support, supervision and guidance from more experienced members of her team to help her; and in addition Sally searched existing literature, extending beyond occupational therapy to help inform her clinical reasoning and practice. She joined the forensic listserve via the internet and posted questions and items for discussions related to her practice.

The team had good resources for patients in terms of both staff and facilities, despite the limitations and constraints of a secure hospital environment. Access to sharp tools and equipment was limited until patients had the appropriate risk assessment and management plans in place.

Joe was beginning to accept the need for help and that there would not be a 'quick fix'. At times he displayed a good sense of humour; the staff on the PDU were cognisant of his needs. He was aware that his personality difficulties had contributed to his index offence – attempted murder – and wanted to explore why. He was trying to avoid self-harm and complying with the risk management plan related to his aggressive and disturbed behaviour.

Stage five – negotiate targeted outcomes and develop action plans

It was important to recognise that Joe had a multi-disciplinary treatment programme which included psychology sessions to explore his offence and personality issues, individual psycho-education sessions with his named nurse, and weekly reviews by the consultant psychiatrist who had prescribed anti-depressant and anxiolytic medicines, sessions with the ward social worker to investigate family issues and possible location of his parents and siblings. There was an ongoing weekly risk assessment and management plans.

Joe and Sally agreed that he needed to start structuring both his day and week in terms of his preferred, potential occupations; therefore they spent time devising a programme of gym, ward-based activities and occupational therapy sessions. She hoped that by participating in occupations and giving Joe choice and opportunities, they would begin to work on his self-esteem, and other intrapersonal difficulties. Both Sally and Joe had considered how his social anxiety would affect his participation. Sally promoted the fact that by addressing his occupational needs this would relate to his criminogenic behaviour.

Stage six – implement plans through occupation

In an attempt to engage Joe in therapeutic activities designed to address his needs, Sally took a measured and graded approach to introduce him to occupational opportunities and enrichment he had never before experienced. She was also aware of the potential risks and management plans which had been identified. Initially they went for walks in the grounds and would have coffee in the patients' social area. Sally encouraged Joe to attend weekly individual gym sessions with a technical instructor. After a while she introduced him to education staff so that he could begin addressing some of his educational needs. Sally provided individual art sessions initially on the ward and then some weeks later they began to use the hospital art room. The eventual aim was to encourage Joe to join a weekly art and pottery group facilitated by a technical instructor.

After many weeks of working with Joe and developing their therapeutic relationship, Sally and Joe were able to address some of his deep-seated difficulties with his self-identity, lack of self confidence and awareness. She was aware that this was going to be a long therapeutic endeavour. Often Joe would lapse into aggressive behaviour and self-harm and his risk management plan would need to change. What was becoming apparent through their sessions was that Joe recognised the need to change his coping and problem-solving skills. Sally worked hard to consider his occupational risk factors and provide opportunities environmentally, socially, and therapeutically. She always used occupations as a medium and introduced Joe to activities he had never had the chance to experience before.

Stage seven – evaluate outcomes

After his initial CPA meeting three months following his admission, Joe's reviews were held every six months. Before each of these meetings Sally and Joe discussed his progress in occupational therapy sessions. They agreed new goals albeit small steps initially. This is often the case with patients such as Joe, a few steps forwards and then some steps back. Given the long-term and entrenched nature of his pathology, Sally had expected this. Nevertheless she persevered with Joe and their therapeutic relationship became stronger and he began to look forward to his occupational therapy sessions. Eventually he had a full weekly programme of therapy, skills and education sessions. He became a member of the hospital football team and became a deputy ward representative. His risks became more manageable and he was able to give an advance directive of what he would like to happen in the event of a violent outburst or episode of self-harming behaviour.

After many months of working with Joe, they began to consider his longer-term needs; this had been too difficult for Joe to do in the earlier stages of therapy. He wanted to develop his work skills so that when he was eventually released and re-integrated into the community he could apply for certain jobs.

Summary

Occupational therapy with patients who have a diagnosis of personality disorder is an exciting and demanding area of forensic practice, with much room for therapeutic optimism. At present there is no significant robust and rigorously tested occupational therapy evidence base about what constitutes best and effective occupational therapy practice.

The purpose of this chapter was to consider how an occupational therapist, in this case Sally, might work in this area without a specific evidence base and how she might overcome this. She was able to use her knowledge of practice and process models to assess, implement and evaluate an occupation-based programme. This began to address some of patient's occupational difficulties. A full multi-disciplinary team approach was necessary to assess the risk, manage and provide him with the extensive treatment he needed to address both his offending behaviour and underlying personality and mental health needs.

This chapter has attempted to demonstrate that occupational therapy can be effective if practitioners consider their underlying occupational therapy knowledge and philosophy, and use the resources available to facilitate occupational enrichment.

References

APA (1994) *Diagnostic and Statistical Manual of Mental Disorders (4th Edition) (DSM-IV)* Washington, DC: American Psychiatric Association.

Baker, S. and McKay, E. (2001) Occupational therapists' perspectives of the needs of women in medium secure units. *British Journal of Occupational Therapy.* **64**: 441–8.

Baron, K., Kielhofner, G., Goldhammer, V. and Wolenski, J. (1999) *Occupational Self Assessment.* Chicago: University of Illinois at Chicago.

Blackburn, R. (1996) Mentally disordered offenders. In: Hollin, C. (ed.) *Working with Offenders: Psychological practice in offender rehabilitation.* Oxford: Wiley.

Blackburn, R., Logan, C., Donnelly, J. and Renwick, S. (2003) Personality disorder, psychopathy, and other mental disorders: co-morbidity among patients at English and Scottish high security hospitals. *Journal of Forensic Psychiatry and Psychology.* **14**: 111–37.

Bonder, B. (2004) *Personality Disorders in Psychopathology and Function*, 3rd edn. Thorofare, NJ: Slack.

Cara, E. (1992) Neutralizing the narcissistic style: narcissistic personality disorder, self-psychology and occupational therapy. *Occupational Therapy in Health Care.* **2–3**: 135–56.

Chacksfield, J. (1997) Forensic occupational therapy: is it a developing specialism? *British Journal of Therapy and Rehabilitation.* **4**: 371–4.

Couldrick, L. (2003) Personality disorders – a role for occupational therapy? In: Couldrick, L. and Alred, D. *Forensic Occupational Therapy.* London: Whurr.

Couldrick, L. and Aldred, D. (2003) *Forensic Occupational Therapy.* London: Whurr.

Crawford, M. (2003) Preface. In: Couldrick, L. and Alred, D. *Forensic Occupational Therapy.* London: Whurr, pp. xv.

Cronin-Davis, J. (2004) Personality disorder. *Therapy Weekly.* **30**: 10.

Cronin-Davis, J. (2005) Disturbed violent behaviour. *OT News.* **13**: 22–3.

Cronin-Davis, J., Lang, M. and Molineux, M. (2004) Occupational science – the forensic challenge. In: Molineux, M. (ed.) *Occupation for Occupational Therapists.* Oxford: Blackwell Publishing, pp. 169–79.

DoH (1990) *HC 90 23/LASL (90) The Care Programme Approach for People with Mental Illness Referred to Specialist Psychiatric Services.* London: HMSO.

DoH and Home Office (1992) *Review of Health and Social Services for Mentally Disordered Offenders and Others Requiring Similar Services, chaired by Dr John Reed. Final Summary Report.* London: HMSO.

Duff, A., Meredith, B. and Woodbridge, K. (2003) *Making Positive Connections.* Brighton: Pavilion.

Duncan, E. (2003) Occupational therapy and the sexual offender. In: Couldrick, L. and Alred, D. *Forensic Occupational Therapy.* London: Whurr.

Duncan, E.A.S. (2006) *Foundations for Practice in Occupational Therapy.* Edinburgh: Churchill Livingstone.

Flood, B. (1997) An introduction to occupational therapy in forensic psychiatry. *British Journal of Therapy and Rehabilitation.* **4**: 375–9.

Forsyth, K., Lai, J. and Kielhofner, G. (1998) *Assessment of Communication and Interaction Skills.* Chicago: University of Illinois at Chicago.

Forsyth, K. and Kielhofner, G. (2005) The model of human occupation: integrating theory into practice. In: Duncan, E.A.S. (ed.) *Foundations for Practice in Occupational Therapy* (4th edn.) Edinburgh: Elsevier Churchill Livingstone.

Fraser, K. and Gallop, R. (1993) Nurses confirming/disconfirming response to patients diagnosed with borderline personality disorder. *Archives of Psychiatric Nursing.* **7**: 336–41.

Hare, R. (1991) *The Hare Psychopathy Checklist-Revised: Manual.* Toronto: Multi-Health Systems.

Hocking, C. (2001) Implementing occupation-based assessment. *American Journal of Occupational Therapy.* **55**: 463–9.

Humphreys, M. (2005) The multi-disciplinary team and clinical team meetings. In: Wix, S. and Humphreys, M. (eds) *Multi-disciplinary Working in Forensic Care*. London: Elsevier Churchill Livingstone, pp. 35–52.

Jones, J. and Plowman, C. (2005) In: Wix, S. and Humphreys, M. (eds) *Multi-disciplinary Working in Forensic Care*. London: Elsevier Churchill Livingstone.

Kielhofner, G. (2002) *Model of Human Occupation*, 3rd edn. Chicago: Lippincott, Williams & Wilkins.

Kielhofner, G., Mallinson, T., Crawford, C., Nowak, M., Rigby, M., Henry, A. and Walens, D. (1998) *A User's Manual for the Occupational Performance History Interview*. Chicago: Model of Human Occupation Clearinghouse.

Lindstedt, H., Söderlund, A., Stålenheim, G. and Sjoden, P. (2004) Mentally disordered offenders' abilities in occupational performance and social participation. *Scandinavian Journal of Occupational Therapy.* **11**: 118–27.

Margolis, R.L. (1996) *Occupational Therapy Task Observation Scale*. Chicago: University of Illinois at Chicago.

Murphy, N. and McVey, D. (2003) The challenge of nursing personality-disordered. patients. *British Journal of Forensic Practice.* **5**: 3–19.

NICE (2005) *The short-term management of violent/disturbed behaviour in psychiatric inpatient and A and E settings*. London: National Institute for Health and Clinical Excellence and National Collaborating Centre.

NIMHE (2003a) *Personality Disorder: No Longer a Diagnosis of Exclusion*. London: Department of Health.

NIMHE (2003b) *Breaking the Cycle of Rejection: The Personality Disorder Capabilities Framework*. London: Department of Health.

Noyes, A. (1955) Personality disorders and their treatments. *American Journal of Occupational Therapy.* **9**: 149–81.

Oxford Dictionary (2005) Available at: http://www.askoxford.com/concise_oed/forensic?view=uk (accessed 29/11/2005).

Quinsey, V., Harris, G., Rice, M. and Cormier, C. (1998) *Violent Offenders: Appraising and Managing Risk*. Washington, DC: American Psychological Association.

Singleton, N., Meltzer, H., Gatward, R., Coid, J. and Deasy, D. (1998) *Psychiatric Morbidity Among Prisoners in England and Wales*. London: TSO.

Stanton, S., Thompson-Franson, T. and Kramer, C. (2002) Linking concepts to a process for organizing occupational therapy services. In: Townsend, E. (ed.) *Enabling Occupation*. Ottawa: CAOT.

Stein, F. and Cutler, S. (2002) *Psychosocial Occupational Therapy,* 2nd edn. Canada: Delmar.

Taylor, C. (2000) *Evidenced-based Practice for Occupational Therapists*. Oxford: Blackwell Science.

Thompson, L., Bogue, J., Humphreys, M., Owens, D. and Johnstone, E. (1997) State hospital survey: A description of psychiatric patients in conditions of special security in Scotland. *Journal of Forensic Psychiatry.* **8**: 263–84.

Thoughts of service users. (2003) In: NIMHE (2003) *Personality disorder: No Longer a Diagnosis of Exclusion*. London: Department of Health.

UKCC (1999) *Fitness for Practice*. London: The UKCC Commission for Nursing and Midwifery Education (Chaired by Sir Leonard Peach). U.K.C. Webster, C., Douglas, K., Eaves, D. and Hart, S. (1997) *HCR-20: Assessing risk of violence (version 2)*. Vancouver: Mental Health Law and Policy Institute, Simon Fraser Institute.

Warren, F., McGauley, G., Norton, K., Dolan, B., Preedy-Fahers, K., Pickering, A. and Geddes, J.R. (2003) *Review of Treatments for Severe Personality Disorder*. Home Office On-line Report 30/03 www.homeoffice.gov.uk/rds/pdfs2/rdsolr3003.pdf (accessed 28/04/2006).

Wester, C., Fraser, S., Douglas, K., Eaves, D. and Hart, S. (1997) Assessing risk of violence in others. In: Webster, C. and Jackson, M. (eds) Impulsivity: Theory, assessment and treatment. New York: Guildford Press.

Whiteford, G. (1997) Occupational deprivation and incarceration. *Journal of Occupational Science, Australia*. **4**: 126–30.

Wilcock, A. (1998) *An Occupational Perspective of Health*. Thorofare: Slack.

Wix, S. and Humphreys, M. (eds) (2005) *Multidisciplinary Working in Forensic Mental Health Care*. London: Elsevier.

Woods, P.R.D. (2002) *The Effectiveness of Nursing Interventions with Personality Disorder*: Manchester: University of Manchester, School of Nursing, Midwifery and Health Visiting.

WHO (1993) *The ICD-10 Classification of Mental and Behavioural Disorders: Diagnostic Criteria for Research*. Geneva: World Health Organization.

Yerxa, B. (2000) Confessions of an occupational therapist who became a detective. *British Journal of Occupational Therapy*. **63**: 192–9.

Further reading

Clarkin, J. and Lenzenweger, M. (eds) (1996) *Major Theories of Personality Disorder*. New York: Guildford.

Young, J. (1999) *Cognitive Therapy for Personality Disorders: A Schema-Focused Approach*. Sarasota, USA: Professional Resource Press.

Livesley, J.W. (2003) *Practical Management of Personality Disorder*. New York: Guildford.

7: Dual diagnosis: learning disabilities and dementia
Working towards ensuring people with a dual diagnosis receive quality services

Mandy Boaz

As stated in *Valuing People: A Strategy for Learning Disability for the 21st Century* (Department of Health (DoH) 2001), people with learning disabilities are more likely to experience mental illness and are more prone to chronic health problems than the general population. In this chapter I will take the reader through my occupational therapy involvement with 45-year-old David and his 78-year-old mother Mary. This will be underpinned by relevant legislation, government initiatives and evidence to support the occupational therapy process. The environment for this chapter will be set within their home and will focus on David who has a diagnosis of Down's syndrome and dementia. People such as David have a high risk of developing dementia and in particular the form known as Alzheimer's disease, with an average age onset of between 30 and 40 years (Prasher and Corbett 1993, Johansson and Terenius 2002). It is important to recognise that there is a paucity of specific occupational therapy literature related to this area of practice. Therefore readers need to be aware that they may well need to draw their evidence base and knowledge from the wider literature.

After reading and reflecting on this chapter the reader should be able to:

- demonstrate an understanding of how Down's syndrome and Alzheimer's disease can affect a person's life;
- explain how legislation and government policy has modernised services for people with learning disabilities;
- reflect on how they could use the occupational therapy process to guide practice when working with a person with learning disabilities.

Historical context of the development of learning disability services

Prior to the nineteenth century the majority of people with learning disabilities in the UK were often cared for in the same hospitals as people with a diagnosis of mental illness. Common terminology used in that period of time included imbecile, mental defective, and moron. With the introduction of new legislation, the Mental Health Act 1959 provided newer definitions, with terminology such as 'mental sub-normality' and 'severe sub-normality' becoming accepted practice (Gates 2004). This act was subsequently replaced with the Mental Health Act 1983 which provided updated terminology to include 'severe mental impairment' and 'mental impairment'.

The highly publicised series of scandals of the 1960s concerning the care of people with learning disabilities in large hospitals in the UK brought about the most significant document of its time, known as *Better Services for the Mentally Handicapped* (DHSS 1971). Key government papers including *Caring for People* (DoH 1989a) and *Working for Patients* (DoH 1989b) began to transform the lives and expectations of people with a learning disability and their families and set in motion the newer models of community-based care.

Wolfensburger (1998) created the concept of normalisation, which refers to people with a learning disability living a normal a life as possible. He further developed this concept into social valorisation, which argued for the need for people to fulfil socially valued roles in society. These important and modernising concepts were captured in the work of O'Brien and Tyre (1981) with what were described as the five service accomplishments. Their work formed the framework for some of today's legislation.

Task box 1

Accomplishments of services (O'Brien and Tyre 1981)

- Community presence
- Choice
- Competence
- Respect
- Community participation

As you read through this chapter try to think of these five accomplishments and see if you can see them reflected in the way practitioners work today.

The Chronically Sick and Disabled Act 1970 came into being, recognising the responsibilities of local authorities to make provision of services to meet the needs of the disabled people including people with a learning disability. The Griffith report (DoH 1988), *Caring for People* (DoH 1989a) and *Working for Patients* (DoH 1989b) resulted in the ground-breaking legislation: National Health Service and Community Care Act 1990. This legislation also transferred the lead responsibilities for the provision of services for people with a learning disability from the

National Health Service (NHS) to local authorities. Local authorities were responsible for developing the care packages of service provision for individuals with a learning disability. This Act still provides the framework for services today. The Disability Discrimination Act 1995, the Human Rights Act 1998, the Carers (Recognition and Services) Act 1995 and the Health Act 1999 provided further legislation that continues to modernise services for all disabled people today.

Several important publications from the Department of Health have contributed to the development of services for people with learning disabilities. You will find it helpful to read these publications, even if you only look at the executive summaries. This will help you develop a deeper understanding of some of the issues that some groups of people have to overcome. The publications are:

The Health of the Nation (DoH 1996) A strategy for people with learning disabilities.

Signpost for Success (DoH 1998) Commissioning and provision of health services for people with learning disabilities.

Once a Day (NHS Executive 1999) A guidance handbook for primary care teams.

Facing the Facts (DoH 1999) A policy impact study of social care and health services.

More recently, the government has published several important documents referred to as national service frameworks. They set out the national standards for services for specific patient and client groups. These publications are also relevant to people with a learning disability. If you go to the Department of Health website (www.doh.gov.uk) you will be able to read about them and see how they apply to people with a learning disability.

The key document for people with a learning disability is the *Valuing People* strategic document (DoH 2001). Why do you think the government decided to develop a strategy rather than a standard setting document? In March 2005 a report of the progress of *Valuing People* (2001) was published. You will be able to see the latest findings from that report at its website (see www.valuingpeople.gov. uk). The main areas of interest related to this chapter are:

Organisations are working better together at a local level.

People are being listened to more.

Person-centred planning, done properly makes a difference to people's lives.

It is preventing people being sent to live away from home.

Further modernisation of services will be carried out for the benefit of people with learning disabilities in the context of the green paper *Adult Services and the Life Chances of Disabled People* (DoH 2005). It would be helpful to you to read this paper.

Before embarking on the referral for David, it is important to have a clear set of principles on which to guide my occupational therapy practice when working with a person with Down's syndrome and Alzheimer's disease. These principles will be complemented by my professional standards of practice (College of

Occupational Therapists (COT 2003) and also the *Codes of Ethics and Professional Conduct* (COT 2005) under which I am able to operate. The principles I have singled out (from Deb 2003) include:

- All interventions should aim to meet the individual's needs to help them remain in their own chosen home and community.
- Caring for a person with Down's syndrome and Alzheimer's disease carries an extra and increasing burden for the family.
- The multi-disciplinary/multi-agency team approach to assessment and service provision which may include care managers and local authority day care and residential staff, general practitioners (GPs), psychologists, nurses, physiotherapists, speech therapists, dieticians and of course occupational therapists will help to lessen the burden.
- The individual and their family need to be known to the community teams for learning disabilities on an ongoing basis.

The occupational therapy process

As previously stated the occupational therapy process provides the structure and organisation to all occupational therapy practice, regardless of client group. It is a guide or in other words a way of working that reflects specific professional standards and codes of practice. Creek (2003) highlights in her definition the importance of collaboration and negotiation to identify problems, and the formulation of goals assist in effective ways of dealing with these problems. Occupational therapy is not unique in using this process but emphasises the importance of occupational performance as being central to therapist's area of concern. This chapter will reflect the occupational therapy process that Creek (2003) describes as encompassing all aspects of treatment implementation and includes 'referral or reason for contact, assessment, problem formulation, goal setting, action planning, action, treatment revision, outcome measurement and discharge' (p. 20).

The referral

I was based within a community team for people with a learning disability and received a direct referral for occupational therapy services for a man named David. He was referred by his designated care manager (from social services) following raised concerns from the local community day centre staff that David was becoming increasingly forgetful and difficult to motivate when participating in his regular weekly activities. David worked in the picture framing/construction section at the day centre and seemed to be having increasing difficulty in completing his tasks. His mother, who was finding it increasingly difficult to manage these changes in his abilities and behaviour at home, had also noted these changes.

David had recently started to have seizures and was under the care and supervision of the family GP. The community nurse for learning disabilities will be mainly involved in the medical interventions and monitoring of this and any other medical problems that David has. If you wish to explore more about epileptic seizures or medical treatments associated with Alzheimer's disease, you will need to access medical and/or nursing textbooks. David and his carer were previously unknown to the community team for learning disabilities. As noted by the commissioners of *Learning Disabilities: The Fundamental Facts* (Emmerson 2001) the majority of people with learning disabilities live in the family home where all too often there is a shortfall of service provision for family carers. Often no plans are made for the future until a family crisis occurs leading to the sudden wrench of emergency residential care for the individual concerned. As noted by Creek (2002) in general, the most positive environment for most people is the home environment.

As part of good practice within the community team all new referrals are shared at the weekly team referral meeting. This is to make sure that a multidisciplinary approach is maintained, enabling the complex needs of people with a learning disability and their carers to receive the most effective service (DoH 2001, Creek 2002). It was agreed that a joint home visit and visit to the day centre with the community learning disability nurse and myself, the occupational therapist would be in the best interests of both David and his mother.

Before meeting David or his carers it was important to have discussions with the care manager who made the referral to the team, so that as much information was gathered and assimilated from different sources as possible. This will enable me to develop an overview of some of the issues that David was currently experiencing. In addition, to be an effective practitioner I will need to have a good understanding of what learning disabilities actually is, what constitutes the diagnoses Down's syndrome and Alzheimer's disease, and how this may impact upon a person's occupational performance.

Definition of learning disabilities

The Department of Health's (2001, p. 4) accepted definition of learning disability is described as follows:

- A significant reduced ability to understand new or complex information, to learn new skills (impaired intelligence) with,
- A reduced ability to cope independently (impaired social functioning),
- Which started before adulthood, with a lasting effect on development.

In this chapter I will use the UK definition of learning disability. The reader will need to be aware that this is not the only definition of the characteristics that have come to represent the term learning disability. It may of interest to the reader to further explore the *International Statistical Classification of Diseases and Related Health Problems* (World Health Organization (WHO) 1994) and the *American*

Diagnostic and Statistical Manual, 4th edition (DSM IV) (American Psychiatric Association (APA) 1994).

David is described on his referral as having an IQ (intelligent quotient) of 50, this would put David in the category of having a moderate learning disability (Rennie 2001). The Department of Health (1992) estimates the prevalence of moderate or severe learning disability to be 3–4 persons per 1000 of the general population. Of these, 70% will have a moderate learning disability. There is much debate about accuracy of the incidence figures; it is not the intention of this chapter to explore this debate, although further investigation into the statistical evidence available from numerous sources may be of interest to the reader.

Selikowitz (1997) suggests that I can expect to see a person who can dress and undress themselves independently/with minimal supervision, wash themselves with minimal supervision, be able to make themselves a simple snack and a hot or cold drink, be able to understand simple instructions and communicate in simple sentences. I anticipate common areas of occupational performance dysfunction with an individual with an IQ of 50 to include activities of daily living.

Outline of Down's syndrome

Down's syndrome is one of the better-known genetic conditions. It is also referred to as a chromosomal abnormality characterised by a specific set of features (Watson 2004). David has been diagnosed with trisomy 21 (presence of three strands of chromosome 21). Some of the main features that David presents with are:

- Small and broad in stature.
- Small round head with a flat face, and with small ears with underdeveloped earlobes. Sparse and thin hair.
- Eyes upward and outward slanting, with an epicanthic fold on the upper lid.
- His nose is small with a poorly developed bridge.
- His mouth often open because he mouth breathes, his tongue appears large and often protrudes from the mouth.
- David wears glasses because he is short sighted.
- David has small hands with short stubby fingers with a distinctive palmar crease.
- David has some speech difficulties and at times can be difficult to understand. He has a stammer and is very quietly spoken so making his needs known can be very difficult for him. Those who know him well can usually understand him and respond to his needs and requests.

Task box 2

Some specific physical features are associated with Down's syndrome. Do you know what these are? In the main text I have named some, you may find it helpful to explore the Down's syndrome association website (www.downs-syndrome.org.uk).

Outline of Alzheimer's disease

In David's case Alzheimer's disease is the second diagnosis that has an impact upon David's occupational performance. It is generally believed that genetic factors are responsible for Alzheimer's disease in adults with Down's syndrome. Other factors, i.e. the environment, may play a part in the development of the condition in later life (Thompson 1999, Temple *et al.* 2001).

Debate continues related to the linking of these two conditions. Past research had discovered localised Alzheimer marker links lying in close proximity to chromosome 21 (St George-Hyslop *et al.* 1987). Although neuropsychological changes may be present in nearly all people with Down's syndrome over the age over 50 years (and markers often present from the age of 30 years) it does not mean that these people will always go on to developing definite signs and deterioration (Post 2002).

Progression of Alzheimer's disease with people with Down's syndrome is quite rapid and aggressive, as is often true of early onset dementia in the main population. Average duration is thought to be about 4.6 years from onset or 4.9–5.2 years (Post 2002). It may be helpful to refer to other chapters in this book to read about the range of clinical features that can affect people with Alzheimer's disease. Post (2002) noted at the top four features affecting people with this dual diagnosis were:

- seizures;
- personality changes;
- apathy/inactivity;
- loss of self-help skills.

The main features affecting David and noted by his carers were: seizures, loss of self-help skills, personality changes (David appeared more irritable and had increased levels of anxiety and memory loss) and forgetfulness. David was observed as becoming increasingly unsteady when he was mobilising. As noted by Rennie (2001) people with Down's syndrome display pre-existing intellectual impairments so that this can lead to a delay in diagnosis adding to the dementia. Thus there is a need for all agencies to work closely with our nursing and medical professional colleagues.

Theoretical models on which I based my practice and interventions with David

It is important to make explicit to the reader the theoretical model that I used to guide my thinking and practice and which seem to best capture the essence of my thinking. The Reed and Sanderson (1999) Human Occupations Model (also known as the Adaptation through Occupation Model) has been developing over the past 20 years. Although described as a process driven, this model purports to the view that occupation is fundamental to human existence as it gives meaning to a person's life. The Reed and Sanderson model is problem based and over the years has become increasingly more client centred. As noted by Hagedorn (2001) the problems are grouped into four areas and include biological, psychological, social and occupational. The main principles are:

- A lack of occupation adversely affects health.
- Occupations become maladaptive.
- Certain occupations hinder adaptation.

Perhaps key to my selection of this adaptation model is that is recognises that sometimes some situations do not always have neat solutions and can be in fact insoluble. In some conditions as in the case of David, with added dilemma of a dual diagnosis, with aggressive deterioration due to Alzheimer's disease, the intervention will focus on the need to minimise the adverse affects of this complex and difficult diagnosis.

The Reed and Sanderson model recognises the importance of the context in which David's performance is set. This includes the environmental context in which David is physically based in the community, his own home and his daily attendance at the day centre. This also takes into consideration the social and cultural environment where David and his Mary his mother are centred. What can be described as temporal aspects of performance directly internally relating to David include the need to consider his age, level of development, his potentially rapidly altering disability status and his life cycle. The Reed and Sanderson model with its basis in occupation guides the practitioner to investigate the performance components as follows:

- sensorimotor components of performance;
- neuromusculoskeletal components of performance;
- cognitive integration of components of performance;
- psychosocial skills components of performance.

Task box 3

I have selected the Reed and Sanderson Adaptation through Occupation Model to guide my thinking and practice. There are many other models that have been developed to assist practitioners, e.g. the Rehabilitative Model (Seidel 2003). Why do you think that I decided not to follow this when working with David?

Approaches to working with David

It is important to identify not only the highly individualised approaches to working with David as a person but also to take into account the approaches recognising the uniqueness of features of Down's syndrome as outlined by Stratford and Gunn (1996). Specific approaches include raising awareness that:

- David will respond better to psychomotor training than to symbol based training

- David's strength of the use of imitation behaviour can expedite his learning the use of gesture when working with David is superior to verbal instruction when learning, e.g. David will imitate me actually walking backwards much more easily than if I ask him to do it
- David will respond better to suggestion than to being directed to complete a task. This is due in part to the tendencies associated with Down's syndrome of drive, impulsiveness and obsessional characteristics
- David's visual processing skills are superior to his auditory processing skills
- David's repetitive tendencies have assisted him to learn tasks through adherence to routines and habit
- David is pressured by time for a speedy response that this will have a direct impact upon the quality of his occupational performance
- David has very poor skills in rehearsing tasks using his working memory, therefore skills take much longer to learn and acquire into tacit knowledge.

This makes working with David together with this dual diagnosis of Down's syndrome and Alzheimer's disease an even more complex challenge. As purported by Creek (2002) it is consistent with both occupational therapy and government policy and guidance that a person-centred holistic approach sits comfortably with this client group (DoH 2001). It is important to see people as a whole and not as an illness and that there is a balance of social, physical and mental health support. This in turn clearly reflects the College of Occupational Therapy *Code of Ethics and Professional Conduct* (2005) which relates to responsibilities and respecting client autonomy in as much as services should be client-centred and needs led.

It is important to include and consider the carer as also one of the central figures to the effectiveness of working with David. In order for David to remain within a home and in his local community environment a client or person-centred approach is imperative to addressing the needs and ongoing support for David and his mother Mary.

The problem solving approach will be utilised with David, which will assist the therapist to look at David's daily routines and occupations and identify areas of difficulty and pursue practical solutions to some of these difficulties. The importance of working with this family in the here and now, in other words dealing with day-to-day issues in the short term is balanced with realistic goals for attainment. The combination of this problem solving approach with the behavioural approach, which uses the therapist's skills in observation, will also guide my practice (Perrin and May 2002).

The behavioural approach (Wilberforce 2004) could be essentially described and demonstrated as elements of behavioural activities or tasks that could be modified and shaped by the use of the reinforcement. In particular that positive reinforcement of particular aspects of behaviour would allow observation of an increase in that particular behaviour. Creek (2002) concurs that positive feedback to encourage both client and carer is essential to its sustained success. Therefore combined with problem-solving which may involve adapting the environment or the way in which David manages the task will provide a practical approach to maintaining and adjusting David's change in skill level of independence. I will also need to consider the role and contribution of the educative approach, particularly when supporting Mary his mother to understand and the pathological course and process that Alzheimer's disease pattern will follow.

Approaches to working with David and his carer

I have focused on a client- or person-centred approach together with a problem solving/ behavioural approach. How might a compensatory approach also have benefited David and his carer?

Assessment

Reed and Sanderson do not specify any particular assessments to complement their developed model of practice so in this instance I have selected assessments that I consider to have meaning and value to the client and their carer.

As noted by Hong *et al.* (2000) many occupational therapists working with people with learning disabilities, mainly use non-standardised assessments. Practitioners note their concerns as to the validity, reliability and robustness of using assessments that are norm-referenced to the general population. In other words comparing one client's performance data with those of another similar client. An argument supported by Plimmer (1996) also supports this view that using standardised assessments with this client group has proved to very difficult in practice. Melton (1996) considered that occupational therapists already used valid assessment tools based upon observations, client and carer interviews and assimilation of pertinent information on which to formulate treatment plans. These were considered to be legitimate methods of occupational therapy assessment. Hagedorn (2001) felt this to be a demonstration of the importance of the humanistic, client-centred values held within the philosophy of occupational therapy. Practitioners may still need to be aware that non-standardised assessments are certainly placed within the lower hierarchy of evidence levels (Muir-Gray 1997).

You may wish to explore the ongoing debate about standardised and non-standardised assessments.

Why do you think that I chose not to use the popular assessment tool Mini-Mental State Examination (Folstein *et al.* 1975) with a person with Down's syndrome?

The Purdue Pegboard (Deb 2003) is used to test the constructional and psychomotor skills of a person. The person has to place as many pegs as they can into round holes on a board within 30 seconds. Why do you think that I chose not to use this popular assessment tool?

Assessments completed with David and his carer

- Initial non-standardised interview
- Pool Activity Level Instrument (PAL) (Pool 2002)
- Assessment of Motor and Processing Skills (AMPS) (Fisher 1995)
- Dementia Scale for Down's syndrome (DSDS) (Gedye 1998)

It may be helpful to familiarise yourself with the above assessments and reflect if you would have chosen them too. If yes why? If not why?

The Canadian Occupational Performance Measure (Law *et al.* 1994) is also a tool that could have been used. Are there any pros and cons of using the tool with David and his mother?

Goal Attainment Scaling (GAS) (Glover and Burns 1994) is a tool to measure the degree to which individualised treatment goals are achieved. Much has been published about this method. Glover and Burns wrote about it in relation to people with severe learning disabilities. Why do you think that I might have chosen not to use this tool?

I used an initial non-standardised interview approach when I first met David and his mother Mary. It was important for me to begin to build a rapport and establish a professional relationship with this family. By sensitive questioning, discussion and observation, this early meeting could be crucial to delivering client-centred, collaborative, effective interventions and services. I felt very much aware that this family might well require a range of ongoing multidisciplinary support as highlighted by Post (2002) because of the aggressive nature of Alzheimer's disease in people with Down's syndrome. The potential duration of the condition of 4.6 years will more than likely be both an emotionally and physically demanding period in their lives.

I used the Pool Activity Level Instrument (Pool 2002) because it is considered to be a user-friendly assessment, specifically designed for people with cognitive impairments based upon carer observation. It involves collaboration between the therapist, the client and the carer and is an aid to establishing an individualised plan, which would be tailored to David's own abilities and needs. The plan therefore is both meaningful and practical and will be identified as part of David's everyday life style. This information includes life history, daily routines, David's abilities and his impairments.

The AMPS assessment (Fisher 1995) is specifically designed for occupational therapists, and to be able to use this assessment tool I had to undergo specialist training. The AMPS was used to assess the underlying motor and performance skills of David's abilities to perform familiar occupations. It was possible to allow David to practise the two to three selected occupations several times before the actual assessment took place. David's choice of familiar occupations included making a sandwich, dressing and potting a plant. Making a sandwich and potting a plant were the more complex and demanding of activities selected. These selected activities were carried out in his own home, familiarity being an essential feature of the assessment. By using the AMPS assessment I was able to determine exactly where and when David was able to perform skills without support and where he needed guidance. The results from the assessment demonstrated that David had marked deficiencies in his processing abilities, this included his ability to search, locate, gather, choose and organise tasks and materials items to carry out the tasks. David had difficulty locating materials and also demonstrated problems using cutlery in the normal manner. His ability to use previous knowledge related to use of familiar objects also showed marked deficiencies and he required cuing to initiate several steps during the activities. David's unsteadiness of gait when moving from one work space to another, including bending, reaching, positioning and stabilising himself was noted. Gathering the results of this assessment information enabled me to make recommendations to his mother and the day care staff. These recommendations included advice regarding modifying and adapting the environment and when staff should assist David in order to be most effective when supporting David during his activities of daily living.

The Dementia Scale for Down's syndrome (Gedye 1998) is one of the most widely used observer-rated scales. To use this assessment specific training is required by the assessor. This assessment lists possible symptoms of dementia at early, middle stages and late stages of the condition. This information provides the therapist and carer with guidelines on the management of symptoms at every stage. This assessment has been described as complex and requires two carers to provide the information separately. The second carer was David's key worker at the day centre where he attends four days per week. The results of this assessment revealed that David was displaying many of the characteristics of mild dementia but more worryingly that scoring reflected some areas within the moderate dementia category.

Problem formulation

Together with the results from the AMPS assessment I was beginning to develop a more comprehensive picture of David's difficulties and problems. The effects of the Alzheimer's disease upon David appeared to be quite extensive and had permeated many aspects of his daily life.

▪ *Forgetfulness.* David was frequently unable to remember family and staff names and could not remember were he put his own belongings, included clothing, bags, books, videos etc.
▪ *Confusion and apraxic symptoms.* From a previously independent dresser David was observed to put clothes on back to front, putting two legs in one trouser and putting two socks on one foot.
▪ *Speech and language problems.* Although David was previously quietly spoken and had a stammer he was now found to engage in repetitive questioning, and was observed to have difficulty following more than one instruction at a time. He had previously been able to use basic Makaton (Walker 1985) signing with speech but he had difficulty remembering some of the hand gestures.

Engaging with David. It now appears increasingly difficult to engage David in activities that were once his main areas of interests. He lacks motivation and has great difficulty finishing any task. David has been observed to become increasingly obsessed on certain aspects of a task and watched the same part of a video over and over again.

Loss of skills – motor and processing skills. As noted in the AMPS assessment his main areas appear to be his processing skills although it was observed that there was some motor skill deficiencies related to unsteadiness when bending and reaching for items. David required more prompts and assistance to complete once familiar tasks. There was also noted to be major slowing down of the pace in all aspects of his motor performance, which is observed as a slowness and increased deliberation in all aspects of his motor performance.

Emotional areas. Emotionally David used to be described as having a placid temperament and a happy personality, keen to be a group member. He appeared less confident in himself and fearful of new experiences. He was now observed engaging in increasingly frequent crying episodes, becoming easily upset and frustrated with himself and other people.

Sleep pattern. David's sleep pattern had become more erratic over the last few months and his mother Mary noted that he was often found wandering around the house in the middle of the night. The community nurse was identified as being the most appropriate health professional to work with this sleep pattern, therefore further exploration of this problem will not be included (Deb 2003).

Epilepsy. As already stated David has recently just started experiencing epileptic seizures and the reader needs to be aware that, with an occurrance of 58% (Post 2002), this was purported to be one of the top problems identified for people with a learning disability and Alzheimer's disease. David had what are described as absences and was receiving medical intervention via his GP. The impact of the epilepsy upon David's functional performance is the main consideration for me, whereas monitoring of seizures and medication is of particular interest to the community nurse for learning disabilities. Practitioners may need to make themselves familiar with the current terminology and treatment for epilepsy.

Risk assessment. The most important consideration for any therapist is the relationship between occupational performance and the need for a comprehensive risk assessment. The occupational therapy service area within the organisation that I work for developed their own specific risk assessment tools which guided my practice. It may also be helpful to explore the Health and Safety Executive website (www.hse.gov.uk).

Think about working with David, what risk assessments you may use/want to use? When and where and how would you carry out risk assessments? Where would you document the results of your risk assessments and who would you share this information with?

Goal setting

My statement for the overall goal of treatment can be summarised as: with the assistance of the multi-agency team, supporting Mary, David to be able to minimise the effects of his ongoing deterioration to meet his changing needs in self-maintenance, productivity and leisure and to achieve satisfaction through occupational and environmental adaptation. In other words: To develop strategies which may assist to support and maintain David's quality of life; and his declining functional skills.

The following performance-related goals as stated by Creek (2003) have to be negotiated, reviewed with agreed priorities set with David and Mary. If they are fully involved throughout the occupational therapy process the greater the likelihood of trust and confidence developing which will aid achievement of these goals. David's dual diagnosis condition and his needs are complex and it must be recognised that it is not practical to expect absolutely every aspect of need to be met. Therefore the necessity for the prioritising of goals is essential. Priority must be based upon what the client/carer sees as the most pressing priority and also the consideration of the major basic underlying problem affecting occupational performance. The main areas for priority goals are agreed as follows:

▓ educative goal;
▓ personal activities of daily living goal;
▓ day centre occupational work goal;
▓ domestic activities goal;
▓ communication/cognitive goal.

Education – goal, plan, action and review

▓ To work with myself, the community nurse, Mary and the key worker at the Day Centre to raise awareness and understanding of impact that Alzheimer's disease has on David's ongoing day-to-day functional ability.
▓ The need for education related to the issues of David having a dual diagnosis of Down's syndrome and Alzheimer's disease. This was actioned through multi-professional joint working between David's GP, the community nurse, the care manager from the adult disabilities team and me. For the day centre staff, a teaching session was organised for all staff that may come into contact with David. This one and half hour teaching session was repeated thrice in order that all the relevant staff were able to attend the session.

Mary his mother already had some awareness and understanding of this dual condition via the Down's Syndrome Association's recent campaigns. Education about the condition that David had developed was a gradual process; this in part was to allow Mary to adjust to this extra burden of care associated with the decreased independence that David was experiencing. Awareness was provided about access to local respite services to allow Mary to have a break from the demands of her caring role (Post 2002). Involvement of social services via David's care manager would enable timely access to local authority occupational therapists.

Looking after a person with a learning disability with high care needs can be an exhausting experience. If you explore www.mencap.org.uk, look for the 2005 publication called 'Breaking Point'. This report evidences the concerns of carers about the lack of respite available for families.

Personal activities of daily living – goal, plan, action and review

To work with David and his carers to maintain and improve his ability to wash and dress himself by simplifying and adapting the tasks.

I will work with David every morning in his own home for one week to establish an appropriate dressing and washing routine and then I will hand this work over to the occupational therapy assistant for a further week. David is undressing currently independently so intervention is unnecessary at the present time. The plan and action is to simplify some of routines and adapt the environment to make the most of his current skills and abilities. Encouraging David to sit down when washing and dressing will make him less vulnerable to falls and help him focus on the task in hand. Gestures and verbal prompts and reassurance will be given to ensure that he washes and dresses correctly. Prompts will be decreased as performance improves. Elements that prove to still cause difficulties or confusion to David will then become part of on going support. Increased time will be given, as this will help him make fewer mistakes when putting on clothes. Clothes will be prepared ready for him to put on, taking into consideration his already established sequencing for dressing. Photographs on doors, cupboards and drawers will assist him to find items that he uses. Once patterns of his performance become more consistent this routine will be returned to his mother Mary to follow. His maintenance and progress will be reviewed with Mary on a regular basis. Advice will also be shared with care manager and staff who will be involved in providing his future respite services.

In the near future David may require the provision of a range of aids and equipment to enable him to remain within the family home. Examples of future adaptive equipment may include grab rails in toilet and bathing areas and provision of a hoist for transfers from bed or bath. It may also be necessary to consider the provision of seating and a wheelchair if his physical condition and abilities deteriorate to assist mobility and access local facilities.

Domestic activities – goal, plan, action and review

To adapt and simplify making snacks and drinks with David, in order for him to maintain his levels of independence.

During the first week I worked on his personal activities of daily living. I will also work him to improve his domestic skills by adapting environments and simplifying tasks. In the kitchen I will use photographs on cupboards to help him find equipment, cutlery and necessary food items so he can find things. Some items used regularly can be set out ready for him to use. The photographs together with cues from me will help David to initiate, sequence and complete tasks. Positive reassurance and guidance will help to reduce his anxieties. He will need to have extra time to complete these tasks if he is to maintain his abilities. Surface areas will need to be free from clutter and extraneous noise distractions removed. Use ready prepared familiar food items, e.g. sliced bread with only what is to be used out to use, sandwich fillings ready to go into the sandwich. Ready to drink cold drinks in bottles or tea already in the teapot and just needs pouring out. There are potentially many activities in the kitchen so it is best to limit how many tasks there are to be completed.

I worked with David to establish routines and then transferred this to the occupational therapy assistant on the second week. The assistant attended every day and during the third week there was a graded handing over period back to his mother Mary. Observation and guidance will be provided and his abilities and skills will be monitored at first on a weekly basis. His ongoing maintenance and progress will be reviewed with Mary on a regular basis. Advice will also be shared with staff from where he attends day care services and may be helpful to future staff in respite services.

Day centre work – goal, plan, action and review

To work with the day centre staff and David to adapt and simplify the picture framing tasks that he is responsible to complete.

My role within the day centre was to work with the staff, rather than working directly with David. This is because their positive contribution and involvement will be central to the continued attendance and maintenance of David at the day centre. Negative staff attitudes towards David would potentially directly affect his performance and behaviour and the quality of experiences (Innes 2002).

I attended the day centre to observe David and the staff working to gain a clearer understanding of the expectations of his role in the picture-framing workshop. I used the same adaptation strategies that were used within his home setting. This included advising staff on reducing extraneous distractions, i.e. clearing work surfaces of unnecessary clutter and equipment. Only having out the tools that he needs to complete the task. Focus on one task to complete only painting one side of picture frames. The use of photographs strategically positioned so that places and items were easier to locate in the building. The importance of allowing more time to complete tasks and move about the day centre building would reduce anxiety for David. I would be making sure that the staff are consistent in their use of gestures, verbal prompts and reassurance when David needs extra support.

The importance of routine, consistency and familiarity was discussed with the staff, including the need to limit staff changes and be increasingly aware of safety issues with equipment. The added issue of David having epileptic seizures in the form of absences will require staff to be extra vigilant and make sure exposure to potential risks are minimised.

Usually a six-monthly review for each service user is carried out at the day centre. In David's case it was thought that a review every two months would seem to be in David's best interest.

Communication and cognition – goal, plan, action and review

As identified and agreed with David and Mary:
◾ To develop a life storybook about David to aid communication, encourage the maintenance of daily routines and as a memory prompt.

As suggested by Gray and Riddon (1999) the importance of developing and maintaining a person's identity gives meaning and purpose to our lives. Life story work was originally used with people with learning disabilities who were leaving old long stay hospitals to live in the community. This communication tool enabled people to be acknowledged and recognised as unique individuals (Bateson *et al.* 2002). A life story book provided detailed information about people's family, friends, likes, dislikes, routines, interests.

David and his mother Mary were keen to do this together and with only minimal advice and guidance, they set about the journey of capturing the life story about David. This goal was client centred and directed by what David wanted in it. This provided an invaluable communication tool so that with David's permission, it was possible for any current or future care staff to gain a better knowledge about David's needs and wishes. The life story book also seemed to give a great deal of personal satisfaction to Mary as she was able to recall many fond memories of their lives together.

Outcome, measurement and evaluation

As I continued to practise in a client-centred way with David and his mother, I was able to realise the importance to this family, of the sharing of the results, outcomes and evaluation of the agreed goals (Creek 2003, Foster 2002). I did not want to overwhelm David and his mother with huge quantities of data therefore decided to limit the tools used in re-assessment and evaluation. I decided to evaluate outcomes of both his personal and domestic activities of daily living with the AMPS assessment tool (Fisher 1995).

David selected the same tasks as he had previously chosen, but had no recollection of the assessment or preparation that we had previously carried out. There were some slight improvements to his previous performance results, which demonstrated to the family that currently, with only minor adaptations, mainly comprising of simplifying tasks, environments, provision of consistent minimal guidance and the use of cues, David had progressed.

The educative and day centre work goals used with Mary his mother and the day centre staff had in part been achieved. Feedback and evaluation was gained through observation and discussion with David, Mary, day centre staff and through the formal multi-agency review meeting process.

Mary and day centre staff were now able to express a greater understanding of the impact that Alzheimer's disease has upon David's current and future skills, abilities and performance. Mary, I felt particularly would continue to need the support and advice from the community nurse. The day centre staff seemed well informed and aware how David could be supported with his work-based tasks. For the staff, issues related to consistency and familiarity of staff members who worked with David, proved more of a challenge to maintain. This would continue to need close monitoring to make sure the effects experienced were minimal upon David.

I believe the most satisfaction and achievement was gained from the use of the life story book. David appeared to gain a great deal of pleasure from collecting items that were of great significance to him. Not only were there photographs of family members and friends but also pictures of where he went to school, the places where he had worked and the local places that he loved to visit. David said that he wanted to make his life story book the biggest book on his bedroom shelf. The family had begun to compile details about David's daily routines, his likes and dislikes. Life story work can be used in an ongoing developmental approach manner, which may take many months to complete.

As David's occupational therapist I strongly believe that the occupational therapy process that I have used was more important than achieving a successful outcome as recognised by Creek (2002), particularly in relation to working with people with deteriorating conditions. The process enabled David to be as independent as was possible and in doing so gaining in confidence, self worth and increased feelings of capability. This gain was observed in both Mary his mother and the day care staff who worked regularly with David.

As opposed to a discharge plan and action, the requirement for ongoing monitoring of his overall well-being and performance needed to continue into the long term. It is likely that interventions will need to be adjusted and adapted as the condition progresses (Finlay 2004). The contribution and involvement of the multiprofessional and multi-agency team will be crucial to the quality of life and level of satisfaction of both David and Mary his main carer.

Conclusion

The purpose of this chapter was to develop the reader's understanding of how a dual diagnosis of Down's syndrome and Alzheimer's disease can affect a person's life, in this case David who was referred to a community team. The chapter provided an historical, social and chronological context about developments for people with learning disabilities on which to base today's working practices.

Specific details relating to both conditions were considered, including exploring the evidence that I used to justify Reed and Sanderson's (1999) 'Adaptation through Occupation Model' and the selected approaches identified. The highly individualised approaches included the person-centred holistic approach, the educative approach to support the main carers, the problem-based approach which clearly complements the overall adaptive model and the behavioural approach to modify and adapt specific elements of David's performance.

The work completed by Stratford and Gunn (1996) recognised specific approaches that were unique and most effective with a person with Down's syndrome and this helped to shape the effectiveness of the occupational therapeutic practice. The professional standards, the code, together with Creek's (2003) interpretation of the occupational therapy process provided the structure on which to guide my interventions.

I have hopefully been able to guide and justify to the reader my selection of assessments, interventions, evaluations and offer opportunities for my opinions and practice to be explored and challenged. Working with David proved to be complex and challenging requiring practitioners, carers and services to work closely together so that David continued to have an acceptable quality of life.

References

APA (1994) *Diagnostic and Statistical Manual of Mental Disorders (4th Edition) (DSM-IV)* Washington, DC: American Psychiatric Association.

Bateson, P., Thorne, K. and Peak, J. (2002) Life story work sees the person beyond the dementia. *Journal of Dementia Care.* May/June: 15–17.

Carers (Recognition and Services) Act 1995. London: HMSO.

Chronically Sick and Disabled Act 1970. London: HMSO.

COT (2003) *Professional Standards of Occupational Therapy Practice.* London: College of Occupational Therapists.

COT (2005) *Code of Ethics and Professional Conduct.* London: College of Occupational Therapists.

Creek, J. (2002) *Occupational Therapy and Mental Health*, 3rd edn. London: Elsevier Science.

Creek, J. (2003) *Occupational Therapy Defined as a Complex Intervention.* London: College of Occupational Therapists.

Deb, S. (2003) Dementia in people with intellectual disability. *Clinical Gerontology.* **13**: 137–44.

DHSS (1971) *Better Services for the Mentally Handicapped.* London: HMSO.

Disability Discrimination Act 1995. London: HMSO.

DoH (1988) *Griffith's Report. Community Care: Agenda for Action.* London: HMSO.

DoH (1989a) *Caring for People.* London: HMSO.

DoH (1989b) *Working for Patients.* London: HMSO.

DoH (1992) *Social Care for Adults with Learning Disabilities* (Mental Handicap LAC) 92 15. London: HMSO.

DoH (1996) *The Health of the Nation. A Strategy for People with Learning Disabilities.* London: HMSO.

DoH (1998) *Signposts for Success in Commissioning and Providing Health Services for People with Learning Disabilities.* London: HMSO.

DoH (1999) *Facing the facts.* London: HMSO.

DoH (2001) *Valuing People: A New Strategy for Learning Disability for the 21st Century.* London: HMSO.

DoH (2005) *Adult Services and the Life Chances of Disabled People.* London: HMSO.

DoH (2005) *The Story so Far – Valuing People.* London: HMSO.

Emmerson, E. (2001) *Learning Disabilities: The Fundamental Facts.* London: Foundation for People with Learning Disabilities.

Finlay, L. (2004) *The Practice of Psychosocial Occupational Therapy*, 3rd edn. Cheltenham: Nelson Thornes Ltd.

Fisher, A.G. (1995) *AMPS Manual.* Fort Collins: Three Star Press.

Folstein, M.F., Forstein, S.E. and McHugh, P.R. (1975) A practical method for grading the cognitive state of patients for the clinician. *Journal of Psychiatry Research* **12**: 189–98.

Foster, M. (2002) Skills for practice. In: Turner, A., Foster M. and Johnson S., (eds) *Occupational Therapy and Physical Dysfunction*, 5th edn. Edinburgh: Churchill Livingstone.

Gates, B. (ed.) (2004) *Learning Disabilities: Towards Inclusion.* London: Churchill Livingstone.

Gedye, A. (1998) *Dementia Scale for Down's syndrome.* Vancouver BC Canada: Gedye Research Consulting.

Glover, S. and Burns, J. (1994) Goal attainment scaling as a method of monitoring the progress of people with severe learning disabilities. *British Journal of Learning Disabilities.* **22**: 148–50.

Gray, B. and Riddon, G. (1999) *Life Maps of People with Learning Disabilities.* London: Jessica Kingsley Publishers.

Hagedorn, R. (2001) *Foundations for Practice in Occupational Therapy.* Edinburgh: Churchill Livingstone.

Health Act 1999. London: HMSO.

Hong, C.S., Smith, N. and Roper, J. (2000). The developments of an initial assessment for people with severe learning disabilities. *British Journal of Occupational Therapy.* **63**: 83–6.

Human Rights Act 1998. London: HMSO.

Innes, A. (2002). The social and political contest of formal dementia care provision. *Ageing and Society.* **22**: 482–99.

Johansson, P.E. and Terenius, O. (2002) Development of an instrument for early detection of dementia in people with Down's syndrome. *Journal of Intellectual and Developmental Disability.* **2**: 325–45.

Law, M. (1994) *Canadian occupational performance measure*, 2nd edn. Toronto: Canadian Association of Occupational Therapists.

Melton, J. (1996) Standardised assessment: people with learning disabilities [letter]. *British Journal of Occupational Therapy.* **59**: 587.

Mental Health Act 1959. London: HMSO.

Mental Health Act 1983. London: HMSO.

Muir-Gray, J.A. (1997) *Evidence Based Healthcare.* Edinburgh: Churchill Livingstone.

National Health Service and Community Care Act 1990. London: HMSO.

NHS Executive (1999) *Once a Day.* London: HMSO.

O'Brien, J. and Tyre, A. (1981). *The Principle of Normalisation: a Foundation for Effective Services.* London: CMH.

Perrin, T. and May, H. (2002) *Well Being in Dementia: An Occupational Approach for Therapist and Carers*, 2nd edn. London: Churchill Livingstone.

Plimmer, L. (1996) Standardised assessments in learning disabilities [letter]. *British Journal of Occupational Therapy.* **59**: 539.

Pool, J. (2002) *Pool Activity Level (PAL). Instrument for Occupational Profiling; a Practical Resource for Carers of People with Cognitive Impairment.* 2nd edn. London: Jessica Kingsley Publishers.

Post, S.G. (2002) Down's syndrome and Alzheimer's disease: Defining a new ethical horizon in dual diagnosis. *Alzheimer's Care Quarterly.* **3**: 215–24.

Prasher, V.P. and Corbett J, A. (1993) Onset on seizures as a poor indicator of longevity in people with Down's syndrome and dementia. *International Journal of Geriatric Psychiatry.* **8**: 923–7.

Reed, K.L. and Sanderson, S.N. (1999) *Concepts of Occupational Therapy*, 4th edn. Philadelphia: Lippincott, Williams & Wilkins.

Rennie, J.C. (ed.) (2001) *Learning Disability. Physical Therapy Treatment and Management.* London: Whurr Publishers.

Seidel, A.C. (2003) Theories derived from rehabilitation perspectives. In: Crepeau, E.B., Cohn, E.S. and Boyt Schell, B.A. (eds) *Willard Spackmans' Occupational Therapy*, 10th edn. Philadelphia: Lippincott, Williams & Wilkins.

Selikowitz, M. (1997) *Down's syndrome the Facts.* Oxford: University Press.

St George-Hyslop, P.H., Tanzi, R.E., Polinsky, R.J. and Haines, J.L. (1987). The genetic defect causing familial Alzheimer's disease maps on chromosome 21. *Science* **235**: 885–90.

Stratford, B. and Gunn, P. (1996) *New Approaches to Down's syndrome.* London: Cassell.

Temple, V., Jozsval, E., Konstantareas, M. and Hewitt, T.A. (2001) Alzheimer dementia in Down's syndrome: The relevance of cognitive ability. *Journal of Intellectual Disability* 45(Part 1): 47–55.

Thompson, S.B.N. (1999) Assessing dementia in people with learning disabilities for cognitive rehabilitation. *Journal of Cognitive Rehabilitation.* **17**: 14–20.

Walker, M. (1985) *Revised Makaton Vocabulary Project*, 4th edn. Camberley: Makaton Vacabulary Development Project.

Watson, D. (2004) Causes and manifestations of learning disabilities. In: Gates, B. (ed.) *Learning Disabilities. Towards Inclusion.* 4th edn. London: Churchill Livingstone.

Wilberforce (2004) Psychological approaches. In: Gates, B. (ed.) *Learning Disabilities. Towards Inclusion.* 4th edn. London: Churchill Livingstone.

Wolfensburger, W. (ed.) (1998). *A Brief Introduction to Social Valorisation: A High Order Concept for Addressing the Plight of Societally Devalued People, and for Structuring Human Services,* 3rd edn. Syracuse, NY: Training institute for human service planning, leadership and change agentry (Syracuse University).

WHO (1994) *International Statistical Classification of Diseases and Related Health Problems,* 10th edn. Geneva: World Health Organization.

8: Working with John Lane: a person-centred approach to supporting the person with dementia and their carers

Caroline Wolverson

This chapter will use the occupational therapy process to integrate theory with practice in relation to John Lane, a 76-year-old man with a diagnosis of vascular dementia. Information relating to John will be introduced throughout the chapter at each stage of the process, illustrating how information is gathered and assimilated in practice. In this way, consideration will be given to ways in which the occupational therapist can contribute to improving services for older people living with dementia using clinical reasoning, the therapeutic relationship and a problem-solving approach (Finlay 2004). Particular attention will be given to the need for effective communication between client, care staff and other agencies. The reader will be encouraged to compare the rhetoric and reality of government policy and be guided throughout this chapter to a range of further reading and tasks. To gain the maximum benefit from this chapter, it should be read in conjunction with Chapter 9.

Objectives

After reading and reflecting on this chapter the reader should have:

- an increased understanding of the experience of someone with vascular dementia living in a residential home;
- considered ways of implementing a person-centred approach when working with a person with dementia;
- developed knowledge of government policy impacting on the lives of older people and the work of therapists.

Government policy

At the 'Improving Care for Older People' Conference (Department of Health (DoH) 2005), the key practical issues involved in improving services and care delivery were discussed. Professor Ian Philp, the older people's tsar, in his presentation 'The NSF: Making Progress', outlined the vision behind the *National Service Framework for Older People* (DoH 2001) as focusing on four key areas:

- Person-centred care
- Joined-up services
- Timely response
- Promoting health and active life

In April 2002, the government introduced national care home standards; these give guidance for both public and private sector organisations to provide best practice. They include service users having their health, personal and social care needs identified in an individual care plan. These standards can support the implementation of interventions by occupational therapists.

Referral information

John, a 76-year-old retired engineer, has been living in a residential care home for the past year following the death of his wife Anne while he was in hospital. John has a diagnosis of vascular dementia and experiences occasional transient ischaemic attacks. He also has arthritis which causes pain and stiffness particularly in his hips and hands. John has one son who lives some distance away and visits his father on a monthly basis.

Staff at the home report that John had become withdrawn over the past three months. They also state that he can be 'uncooperative' with personal care tasks and has been verbally aggressive towards residents. John's mobility had deteriorated to the extent that he required a wheelchair when outside of the home. He is incontinent of urine at times, which staff considered to be 'attention seeking'.

The referral was presented at the weekly community mental health team meeting where it was decided that the community psychiatric nurse would carry out an initial assessment. She requested a joint visit with the occupational therapist.

A person-centred approach (see Task box 1)

Standard Two of the *National Service Framework for Older People* (DoH 2001) focuses on person-centred care, its aim being

> *'To ensure that older people are treated as individuals and they receive appropriate and timely packages of care which meet their needs regardless of health and social services boundaries.'*

Kitwood (1997) stated that the person-centred approach of working emphasised communication and relationships, while Brooker (2004) suggests it means different things to different people: to some a value base and to others individualised care. Drawing on previous work by Kitwood, she identifies person-centred care as encompassing four main elements:

- valuing the person and those who care for them;
- treating people as individuals;
- looking at the world from the perspective of the person with dementia;
- providing a positive social environment in which the person can experience relative well-being.

Task box 1: Enhancing person-centred care

To provide person-centred care it is necessary to know as much about the person as possible. Knowledge of vascular dementia will inform you of how the condition might present in a person but how can you begin to understand the subjective experience of dementia? Berenbaum (2005) suggests the following:

- Read accounts written by people with dementia, for example *Who will I be when I die?* by Christine Astley Boden (2004) and *My Journey into Alzheimer's Disease* by Robert Davis (1989)
- Listen carefully to what the person is saying to you during assessment and interventions
- Listen carefully and imaginatively to what people say in the normal course of life
- Observe behaviour and actions
- Speak to those who have recovered from dementia-type illnesses
- Use your poetic imagination
- Using role play with colleagues

Assessment

Assessment is a means of gathering relevant information to inform the prioritisation and development of goals. It is also a means of measuring change and evaluating interventions (Duncan 2006). When considering assessment with John, it is important to take into account the components of person-centred care as identified by Brooker (2004): valuing John and those who care for him, treating him as an individual and looking at the world from his perspective. Consideration also needs to be given to whether others are treating him in this way and if he is living in a positive social environment.

To assess and work with John effectively it is essential to establish a therapeutic relationship. The therapist needs to acknowledge that this requires time, especially when working with someone with dementia who may not remember previous contacts or what has been said earlier in the conversation.

Task box 2: Establishing a therapeutic relationship

Given the information from the case study, what challenges might there be in establishing a therapeutic relationship with John? How can you work to overcome these?

Recommended reading:

- Bonham, P. (2004) *Communicating as a Mental Health Carer*. Cheltenham: Nelson Thornes.
- Creek, J. (2002) *Occupational Therapy and Mental Health*, 3rd edn. Edinburgh: Churchill Livingstone.
- Finlay, L. (2004) *The Practice of Psychosocial Occupational Therapy*, 3rd edn. Cheltenham: Nelson Thornes.
- Goldsmith, M. (2002) *Hearing the Voice of People with Dementia; Opportunities and Obstacles*. London: Jessica Kingsley Publishers.
- Powell, J. (2000) *Care to Communicate: Helping the Older Person with Dementia*. London: Hawker Publications.

Perrin and May (2000) advocate an assessment process that results in positive engagement and improving well-being. The assessment process began before meeting John, with the information gained from the referral letter. As the process continued, information was gathered from a range of sources but most importantly from John himself. Task box 3 lists a range of assessment methods. Remaining person-centred is crucial, this means choosing each assessment tool carefully and not over assessing. It is important to draw on information that has previously been gathered so as to reduce repetition for John. The Single Assessment Process (DoH 2001) would have enabled this as it covers a range of general issues and thus serves to reduce duplication. It is also important to have John's consent to gather information from other sources.

Task box 3: Assessment

Perrin and May (2000) identify a number of possible assessments to use with people with a diagnosis of dementia – see below. Consider why you might use each.

- Allen's leather lacing assessment (Allen 1990). Functional leather lacing task to identify the person's cognitive level ranging from level 1 (automatic actions) to level 6 (planned actions).
- Dementia Rating scale (Psychological Assessment Resources 1998). Assesses cognitive capacity and provides insight into why the person may be experiencing difficulties with engagement.
- Functional Performance Profile (Mullhall 1993). Recording observable actions and behaviours in a range of different areas.
- Dementia Care Mapping (Kitwood and Bredin 1992). Records the nature and quality of engagement experienced by people who have dementia and levels of well-being.

A further relevant assessment is the Assessment of Motor and Process Skills (Fisher 1997) which is a standardised observational assessment offering the opportunity to simultaneously evaluate the person's ability to perform personal and domestic or instrumental activities of daily living and the quality of their motor and process skills. To use this assessment, the assessor must be trained in its use.

What are the benefits of using standardised and non-standardised assessments with John?

Assessment process

Informal Interviews

Informal interviews were conducted over several meetings with John as his concentration was limited. Consideration was given to John's capacity to engage in the interview process; ensuring that he was given time to respond to questions and was not overloaded with too much information. In order to put John at ease, an informal manner was adopted and open-ended questions used. Engaging John in conversation was another means of gathering information and helped to build a relationship. In addition some closed questions were used as these were sometimes easier for John to process and respond to. A semi-structured format ensured that all necessary areas were covered. An interest checklist was also used; containing both pictures and words in order to enable John to participate more fully. Overall, however, it was essential that time was taken to learn how to communicate well with John. Pitkin (2004) states that if professionals really wish to demonstrate their understanding of person-centred care then acquiring sensitive communication skills and gathering a detailed personal history of the person is imperative.

Observation

It is important to remember that observation does not only relate to John directly. From the moment of entering the home environment and meeting the care staff, assessment of John's physical and social environment began, as both may have contributed to the changes in his behaviour (Stokes 2002). Observation of John at different times of the day was also necessary to assess specific tasks and take account of fluctuations in function throughout the day.

During interactions with John, consideration was given to indicators of well-being such as a relaxed posture, sense of humour, alertness and responsiveness (Bruce 2000). Careful listening to the messages behind what was being said and observation of body language also helped to provide information about John's feelings which he may not have been able to express verbally.

The Pool Activity Level (Pool 2002) is an example of an observational tool which may be used to gather assessment information. Pool (2002) states that this instrument draws on several models of understanding human behaviour: the lifespan approach to human development; dialectical model of a person-centred approach (Kitwood 1997); and the cognitive disability model (Allen 1985). The Pool Activity Level is based on the principle that people with cognitive impairment have potential abilities that can be realised when in an enabling environment; and that occupation is the key to unlocking this potential. Pool (2002) recommends that several of those involved in the person's care complete the checklist to identify variation in ability over a period of time. The results on completion of the checklist will identify an activity level at which John is able to work at and assist in implementing activities at an appropriate level to encourage success.

Although assessments with John were not standardised (informal semi-structured interview and observation) and therefore lacked the reliability of more standardised assessments, Keilhofner (2002) identifies the following as some of the reasons to support their use:

- lack of time to complete structured assessment;
- unacceptability of assessment by client;
- lack of appropriate structured assessments.

It could be argued that that these were not sufficient reasons for the lack of use of standardised assessments. However, it was felt initially that the priority was to establish a therapeutic relationship with John and while doing this, assessment information was able to be gathered in an informal way which was acceptable to John.

Joint visit by occupational therapist and community psychiatric nurse

On meeting with John in his room at the care home, he was unshaven and his glasses were in need of cleaning. John was sitting quietly, but appeared pleased to have visitors and was willing to talk with us. His room had few personal belongings other than a radio which was not switched on and a framed photograph of himself and his wife. He initially responded to questions but after about 15 minutes became tired and agreed to us visiting a couple of days later. Names, contact numbers and an appointment card were left with him. On the next visit, John had remembered our names, although he had forgotten that we were visiting on that day. On this occasion, he was more animated but again tired quickly and expressed discomfort from sitting for a long period in his chair.

As it was near lunchtime, I stayed and walked with John to the dining room and with his agreement, stayed with him over lunch. From this point the community psychiatric nurse and I agreed to visit separately but shared information with each other after each visit.

When discussing John with care staff, they reported that he frequently put soiled clothes on top of clean ones in his wardrobe, and had attempted to hit another resident on two previous occasions. It became apparent that staff had developed an unhelpfully negative attitude towards John, which the manager of the home was keen to address. A further example of this was stating in the referral information that John was aggressive towards other residents. On further questioning of staff and John, it was found that he had been verbally aggressive towards one resident. This was a gentleman with dementia who repeatedly entered John's room and whom John stated that he was fearful of. The first step towards addressing the negative attitude of staff was the appointment of a new key worker for John.

During these initial visits, John expressed an interest in spending time away from the home and so the next visit was arranged with a view to accompanying him to the nearby park. John required a wheelchair as his mobility was limited due to pain and stiffness arising from arthritis. Away from the home, his mood appeared to lift. His conversation was more animated, his concentration improved and he took an active interest in his environment. The session lasted approximately one hour and he was able to concentrate throughout.

Care planning

Results of assessment

The initial assessment phase took place over a two-week period and involved four visits from the occupational therapist. This included an early morning visit to assess John with dressing and washing as at this time staff were providing full assistance which John did not feel he needed. Assessment by the nurse had included completion of the Mini-Mental State Examination (Folstein *et al.* 1975) and the Hospital Anxiety and Depression scale (Zigmund and Snaith 1994), which, in addition to talking with John, had suggested that he was depressed. A referral was made to the psychiatrist to discuss with John the management of his depression. A request was made to his general practitioner (GP) for physical health screening, to discuss medication to assist with pain management for arthritis, and to investigate the cause of John's urinary incontinence. John was found to have a urine infection for which he was prescribed antibiotics. This illustrates the importance of investigating any changes in behaviour and not simply attributing them to cognitive impairment. Consideration needs to be given to physical health, past history, and the social and physical environment; all of which may impact on the person's behaviour (Stokes 2002).

From talking with John and his carers, observing him within his home environment, completing an interest checklist and working with care home staff to complete the Pool Activity Level, a treatment plan was devised to address key areas of difficulty for John. As a result of the difficulties identified, his level of well-being and quality of life were reduced. He rarely showed signs of well-being, such as relaxed posture and sense of humour and frequently presented with signs of ill-being such as being withdrawn, anxious and an inability to communicate his needs (Bruce 2000).

John's identified long-term goal

To improve quality of life and well-being.

An overview of areas of difficulty and related short-term goals can be seen in Tables 8.1–8.5.

Table 8.1 Personal care.

Identification of problem area	▪ Lack of opportunity for independence in personal care – at present fully assisted in this at variable times each morning ▪ Becomes embarrassed when incontinent therefore puts soiled clothes in wardrobe ▪ Staff frustrated by John doing this and have removed all clean clothes from wardrobe – also believe that incontinence was purposeful to get attention
Translate to needs	**Problem re-framed** ▪ John would like to get up at a regular time of his choosing and have the opportunity to manage his own personal care needs with support
Identify strengths	▪ John has previously been a smart and tidy person taking pride in his appearance ▪ John is able to function at a planned activity level (Pool 2002) – working towards completing a task but may not be able to solve problems that arise during task ▪ During assessment John had demonstrated his ability to be independent in personal care tasks with visual and verbal prompts ▪ John is a private man who wishes to be as independent as possible
Realistic goal	**To improve routine and management of personal care** ▪ Staff to assist John to put out his clothes for the next day each evening ▪ John provided with alarm clock which staff help to set for 7 am each day ▪ Prompt given at 7.15 an each morning for John to get up and washed ▪ Step by step guide for John placed in clear view in his room to prompt him with washing and dressing ▪ Discussion with care staff with regard to the causes of John's incontinence and formulation of strategy – clothes returned to wardrobe, labelled laundry basket provided in room, staff to prompt John regularly to go to the toilet

Prioritisation of need

Using a person-centred approach it is important to prioritise the goals which John wishes to achieve first, however, this must be balanced with risk. For example with John there is a danger of his health and well-being being adversely affected by the negative attitudes towards him on the part of the home care staff. Working with staff in order to overcome these attitudes would also be seen as a priority, although not necessarily by John. Goals with a relatively easy solution may also be considered initially as these would give a quick result and help John to feel positive towards engagement with the service (Finlay 2004).

Table 8.2 Independence in chosen occupations.

Identification of problem area	John's physical and cognitive difficulties in addition to his environment have resulted in a lack of confidence, control and opportunity to engage fully in chosen occupations
Translate to needs	**Problem re-framed** John would like to be more confident and independent in his daily routine and chosen occupations
Identifying strengths	John is able to function at a planned activity level (Pool 2002) therefore will be able to make use of equipment and prompts if given clear instructions

Realistic goal	**To improve independence and opportunity to engage in purposeful occupations and develop daily routine**
	  Assessment and provision of walking stick to aid mobility
	  Provision of large grip cutlery to improve function and reduce pain at meal times
	  Provision of daily planner in clear view in bedroom
	  Provision of large clock in clear view in bedroom
	  Provision of clear labels and pictures within the home to aid orientation, for example on bathroom doors
	  Provide name and picture on bedroom door
	  Provide key to room to help John feel ownership and prevent other residents entering room (John was particularly fearful of a gentleman with severe dementia who repeatedly entered his room – he had responded with verbal aggression)
	  Provision of window bird feeder and hanging baskets. John to be involved in preparation and maintenance of these

Table 8.3 Life story book.

Identification of problem area	John has limited opportunity for purposeful occupation, a lack of routine and control in his life, and is supported by people who have a negative attitude towards him
Translate to need	**Problem re-framed** John would like to engage in more purposeful occupations and have opportunity to be creative. He would like staff to know him better and have a more holistic care plan. This would give opportunity to feel valued and in doing so increase well-being and self-esteem

Identify strengths	John is able to function at a planned activity level (Pool 2002)
	  John will benefit from an activity that has a clear end product
	  John has good recognition of faces and names
	  John has travelled widely and has an interest in local history
	  John has a wide range of interests
	  John has previously enjoyed socialising

Realistic goal	**To develop a life story book to encourage focus on previously enjoyed activities and present needs**
	  Sessions to take place twice weekly over four weeks initially using photographs as a starting point
	  Involvement of key worker to help John record his memories
	  Involvement of son to bring familiar possessions to decorate John's room
	  Agreement to this being shared with care staff. It is essential that permission is always gained from the client for sharing of information (COT 2005)

Table 8.4 Community-based activities.

Identification of problem area	John has a lack of opportunity for friendship and socialisation; he is socially excluded
Translate to need	**Problem re-framed** John would like to take part in community activities and have opportunity to socialise and develop friendships
Identify strengths	▫ John has enjoyed being part of a range of social groups ▫ John has good social skills and is able to communicate effectively when feeling well
Realistic goal	**To encourage social inclusion through community based activities** ▫ Provision of befriender to accompany John to local history group and visits to the pub ▫ Staff to encourage John to engage in activities and trips within the home

Table 8.5 Staff training.

Identification of problem area	John has no meaningful relationships with people around him. He is cared for by staff who have a negative attitude towards him and a lack of knowledge about dementia
Translate to need	**Problem re-framed** The manager of the home recognises that staff lack knowledge and understanding to care for John effectively
Strengths	▫ John does not wish to move to a new home ▫ There is a new home manager who is keen to implement change ▫ John has a new key worker whom he is beginning to establish a positive relationship with
Realistic goal*	**To provide staff training sessions to encourage increased knowledge for dementia and of John as a person** ▫ Provision of three staff training sessions over a one month period ▫ Provision of additional support when required ▫ Provision of information booklet for staff ▫ Six month review and evaluation

*Although this goal is therapist led, John remains at the centre of this goal.

When working with John to achieve his goals it is necessary to consider ways to maximise engagement. This can be done through (Powell 2000, Goldsmith 2002):

▫ giving choice;
▫ providing opportunity for emotional outlet;
▫ including a sensory experience;
▫ building on previously enjoyed activities;

- providing opportunity for relaxation and pleasure;
- selecting a time of day best suited to John;
- giving time to work at John's pace.

Consideration must also be given to working in an ethical way (*Code of Ethics and Professional Conduct*, College of Occupational Therapists (COT) 2005), see Task box 4.

Task box 4: Ethical issues

Throughout our work with John we must consider ethical issues. Some of these might be:

- Consent
- John's capacity to make decisions
- Confidentiality
- Empowerment
- Human rights
- User involvement
- Power
- Choice
- Risk

How might these impact on working with John? Further reading:

- Cheston, R., Bender, M. and Byatt, S. (2000) Involving people who have dementia in the evaluation of services: a review. *Journal of Mental Health.* **9**: 471–9.
- COT (2005) *Code of Ethics and Professional Conduct.* London: College of Occupational Therapists.
- Faulkner, M. (2001) Empowerment, disempowerment and the care of older people. *Nursing Older People* **13**: 18–20.

Evidence to support interventions

To improve routine and management of personal care (see Table 8.1)

Sacco-Peterson and Borell (2004), Chung (2004) and Ballard *et al.* (2001) have demonstrated that participation in self-care can contribute to health and well-being. This is often a challenge for people within the care setting, as identified by Sacco-Peterson and Borell (2004) in their study of a nursing home ward. They found that residents had to overcome greater physical and cognitive challenges to maintain their participation and autonomy in personal care tasks than if they were living at home.

The Alzheimer's Society identifies the importance of encouraging a regular routine to maintain function and well-being. Findings of *The Literature and Policy Review into Mental Health and Well-being in Later Life* (Seymore and Gail 2004) also suggest a positive link between routine and mental health.

To improve independence and opportunity to engage in purposeful occupations, and develop a daily routine

Studies have demonstrated that a person's need for purposeful activity is preserved throughout life (Lansdown 1994, Perrin 1997). Green and Cooper (2000) used the Person-Environment-Occupation Model (Law *et al.* 1996) to assist in organising a study entitled 'Occupation as a quality of life constituent: a nursing home perspective'. This model can be used to identify the strengths and problems with occupational performance and addresses the importance of the relationship between environment and the person's level of occupation. It proposes that the relationship is dynamic and interwoven. Law *et al.* represent this by three inter-related circles. Where the circles overlap occupational performance is achieved. In Green and Cooper's study of 20 nursing homes they found that it was necessary to have a flexible environment and wide interpretation of occupations to facilitate quality of life. Volicer *et al.* (2000) highlight the importance of the occupations of people with dementia not just being limited to organised activity; there should be the opportunity to engage in all aspects of activities meaningful to them and related to their roles. Chung (2004) in her study of 62 nursing home residents describes an example of encouraging enjoyment and pleasure at mealtimes rather than the focus being on the person finishing their food. In John's case, his well-being and quality of life were improved through physical and social changes being made to the environment and adaptations and compensatory techniques being used to increase his opportunity for independence and engagement in his chosen occupations. Examples of this were the sensory experience he received from watching birds at his window and listening to music.

As can be seen from Table 8.2 a range of equipment such as a walking stick and large grip cutlery were provided to aid independence. In this way, John's confidence was increased in mobilising and pleasure at meal times was increased. Adaptations to the environment such as labelling rooms and providing a daily planner again contributed to increased independence. John was supported in learning to use these and this was maintained through continued prompts from staff. Instructions for staff on how to do this were incorporated into his care plan.

Life story book: Engagement in purposeful occupation (Table 8.3)

Murphy (1994) describes life story work as looking back on the past but not setting out to resolve past or present problems although he acknowledges that this may be an outcome. The Cochrane Review of reminiscence therapy for dementia by Wood *et al.* (2005), aims to consider the effects of reminiscence therapy on people with dementia and their care-givers. The review found that the evidence base for reminiscence therapy rests mainly on descriptive and observational studies, with the few randomised control trials available being small and of relatively low quality. They do, however, acknowledge its popularity with staff and participants and found that staff knowledge of participants' backgrounds increased dramatically in comparison with those who did not receive the intervention. This increased knowledge can only serve to improve care planning, person-centred care and through this, well-being for the individual.

Clouston (2003) describes life story as being a valuable tool through which service users can be heard, are able to participate actively and through this, be empowered. Developing a life story book with someone offers a person-centred activity giving opportunity to value the person and look at the world from their perspective. This is confirmed by Goldsmith (2002) who states that through understanding of a person's past we can better understand their present situation.

A study by Batson *et al.* (2002) identified one of the benefits of being involved in gathering information for life story books is that it helps the gatherer to have greater knowledge of the person for whom they are caring and helps them to see beyond the condition. This was confirmed by Clarke *et al.* (2003) who found that collaboration between carers, staff and clients to develop a biographical profile enhanced relationships between them in having a positive effect on attitudes and increasing personhood of the person with dementia. A further perspective is offered by Murphy (1994) cited in Goldsmith (2002) who highlights the value of the process rather than the end product, recognising the importance of the person wishing to share. Another benefit of life story work is the opportunity for creativity which Perrin (2001) views as being central to the order of human life.

Task box 5: What is a life story book?

When suggesting an intervention to a person, it is useful to have had experience of this yourself. Consider your own life story thinking about significant events in your life and the people who are important to you. Also, what would be important for others to know, if you were no longer able to communicate effectively. You may want to write these thoughts down, or collect images or photographs that represent your thoughts.

What are the potential challenges to creating a life story book with someone and how would you work to overcome these?

This chapter gives you information and references to develop your knowledge of life story work.

To encourage social inclusion through community-based activities

The importance of maintaining John's improved mood was essential to his continued health and well-being. Previously, John had little opportunity to engage in past hobbies such as local history and music and limited opportunity for meaningful relationships. Working with John to achieve his goals, it was important to consider how these could be maintained when the period of occupational therapy intervention was complete. One way was to involve other agencies to enable John to have an established routine to his leisure time and give him opportunity to engage in previously enjoyed activities.

The Government drive is to implement a strategic partnership between the NHS, voluntary and community sector. Traditionally people in residential homes have often been denied the opportunity to engage in community services as it is assumed that their needs will be met by the care home, however, this can lead to social exclusion. As occupational therapists it is necessary to have excellent networking skills; to be aware of local agencies and services which people can utilise; have good links with those who work in these services and know how to assist people to engage with them.

Befriending service

This provided John with a valuable social outlet that was not connected with the home and provided contact with the local community. Greenberg *et al.* (1999) in their study of a support group for older women, identified the importance of friendship contributing to positive mental health. This is supported by a qualitative study by Hedelin and Strandmark (2001) who found the involvement in one's relationships to oneself and others was one of the components of positive mental health. Although these studies are of women, it could be argued that they are transferable to John's experience as can be demonstrated by his continued improved mood and desire to maintain these contacts. Okum *et al.* (1984) and Menec (2003) found a positive relationship between social activity and well-being.

Voluntary agencies

The local Age Concern provided a variety of activities including concerts and music events which it was thought, given John's previous interest in music and theatre, would be a positive experience for him. On discussion with John, he stated that he did not wish to do this as it was an interest that he had shared with his wife and he would find it too upsetting to attend these without her at this time. It is important to remember that just because someone has previously enjoyed an activity does not mean that they will continue to do so when circumstances change. John still enjoyed listening to music and with the help of his key worker, he purchased a CD player for his room.

For provision of staff training sessions to encourage increased knowledge for dementia and of John as a person, see Task box 8.6.

The assessment of John and his home environment identified negative staff attitudes towards him. Their understanding of dementia was poor and they felt that John was presenting with challenging behaviour to seek attention. It was therefore crucial to his well-being that the community mental health team worked with staff using an educative approach to teach them about working with people with dementia and also specifically to encourage them to work positively with John and find out about the 'person behind the dementia' (Batson *et al.* 2002).

When considering staff training, I was aware that staff needed to be provided with training if they were to provide quality care, but at present this often focuses on training in basic physical care (Innes 2002). Lack of staff training to increase understanding and knowledge of working with people with dementia will again serve to make staff feel disempowered and undervalued particularly when faced with difficult situations of which they have limited knowledge of how to respond. The undervaluing and low status of care staff can often be seen to mirror attitudes to people with dementia.

On completion of the formal staff training it was important to maintain a good working relationship with the home manager and care staff and continue to provide them with support when necessary. It was essential to develop and maintain good communication systems which enabled them to feel supported and comfortable in seeking advice. In addition, follow-up training sessions were provided to maintain the improved knowledge and approach of staff.

Time was also spent with the newly appointed activity co-ordinator to discuss the use of activity in the home to best meet peoples' needs. With support of the home manager she was encouraged to join the National Association of Providers of Activity for Older People (NAPA) which has recently launched a strategic partnership with the College of Occupational Therapists to promote occupational opportunities for older people, particularly in care homes.

Task box 6: Implementation of staff training

■ How might you implement this to achieve the best results?
■ How would you evaluate the success of staff training?

Suggested reading:

■ Bryan, K., Axelrod, L., Maxim, J., Bell, L. and Jordan, L. (2002) Working with older people with communication difficulties; an evaluation of care worker training. *Aging and Mental Health.* **6**: 248–54.
■ Davies, K., Lambert, H. and Turner, A. (2005) Training for care staff. *Journal of Dementia Care.* **13**: 18.
■ Perrin, T. (ed.) (2004) *The New Culture of Therapeutic Activity for Older People.* Bicester: Speechmark Publishing Ltd.
■ Sheard, D. (2005) Training with heart. *Journal of Dementia Care.* **13**: 5.

Evaluation

Evaluation is integral to the occupational therapy process. Traditionally the involvement of people with dementia in evaluation of the service they receive has been limited, often relying on evaluation by carers. In considering evaluation with John, several methods could be used:

  review of achievement of goals with John;
  undertaking a satisfaction questionnaire with John;
  repeat of assessments used; for example the Hospital Anxiety and Depression Scale (Zigmund and Snaith 1994);
  observation of increased signs of well being such as communicating wants, needs and choices, showing pleasure and enjoyment (Bradford Dementia Group 2002);

feedback from care staff;

personal reflection on work with John.

Brooker and Duce (2000) states that the maintenance and improvement of wellbeing in people with dementia is the therapeutic outcome indicator that best fits with current psycho-social models of dementia care. As an occupational therapist working with other members of the multi-disciplinary team it will be important to review and reflect on involvement with John as a team. Evaluation will also take place at the review meeting for John within the home.

Conclusion

Involvement with John took place over a two-month period. During this time, with the involvement of the community mental health team, his mood gradually improved and his independence and well-being increased. At this time, his life story book was completed, he had a regular routine established and he was again involved within the home and local community. As the goals of treatment had been met, it was agreed with John and the community mental health team that I would discharge him. The community psychiatric nurse continued to monitor John's mood and cognitive function in addition to supporting staff within the home. Where necessary, discussion would take place within team meetings with regard to John's mental health and well-being and there was the opportunity for re-involvement if necessary.

This chapter has aimed to develop the reader's knowledge of working with someone with dementia using a person-centred approach. Assessment and interventions have involved the use of clinical reasoning, problem-solving and reflection to consider John's lived experience and to work with him and the care home staff to improve his quality of life and well-being. Attention has been given to working in collaboration with members of the community mental health team and the care staff to encourage a cultural shift within the home, enabling the staff to know John and value him as a person. The four key areas of focus in the *National Service Framework for Older People* (DoH, 2001) have been considered throughout: a person-centred service with links across agencies, providing a timely response for John and one which promotes health and an active life. It is only through effective communication, collaboration and taking time to get to know the person that we can truly be person-centred and effective in enhancing quality of life and well-being.

References

Allen, C.K. (1985) *Occupational Therapy for Psychiatric Diseased: Measurement and Management of Cognitive Disabilities.* Boston: Little, Brown.

Allen, C.K. (1990) *Allen Cognitive Test Manual.* Colchester: S and S Worldwide.

Astley Boden, C. (2004) *Who will I be when I Die?* Australia, HarperCollins.

Ballard, C., O'Brien, J., James, I., Mynt, P., Lana, M., Potkins, D., Reichelt, K., Lee, L., Swann, A. and Fossey, J. (2001) Quality of life for people with dementia living in residential and nursing home care: The impact of performance on activities of daily living, behavioural and psychological symptoms, language skills and psychotropic drugs. *International Psychogeriatrics.* **12**: 93–106.

Batson, P., Thorne, K. and Peak, J. (2002) Life story work sees the person beyond the dementia. *Journal of Dementia Care.***10**: 15–17.

Berenbaum, R. (2005) Learning about the lived experience of dementia. *Journal of Dementia Care.* **13**: 20–1.

Bradford Dementia Group (2002) *Well-being Profiling.* Bradford: University of Bradford.

Brooker, D. (2004) What is person-centred care? *Clinical Gerontology.* **12**: 215–22.

Brooker, D. and Duce, L. (2000) Well-being and activity in dementia; A comparison of group reminiscence therapy, structured goal-directed activity and unstructured time. *Aging and Mental Health.* **4**: 354–8.

Bruce, E. (2000) Looking after well-being: a tool for evaluation. *Journal of Dementia Care.* **8**: 25–7.

Chung, J. (2004) Activity participation and well-being of people with dementia in long-term care settings. *Occupational Therapy Journal of Research.* Winter **24**: 22–31.

Clarke, A., Hanson, E. and Ross, H. (2003). Seeing the person behind the patient: Enhancing the care of older people using a biographical approach. *Journal of Clinical Nursing.* **12**: 697–706.

Clouston, T. (2003) Narrative methods: talk, listening and representation. *British Journal of Occupational Therapy.* **66**: 136–41.

COT (2005). *Code of Ethics and Professional Conduct.* London: College of Occupational Therapists.

Davis, R. (1989) *My Journey into Alzheimer's Disease.* Illinois: Tyndale House Publishers.

DoH (2001) *National Service Framework for Older People.* London: The Stationery Office.

DoH (2005) Improving Care for Older People Conference 2005 [online] Available from: www.dh.gov.uk/NewsHome/ConferenceAndEventReports/ConferenceReportsConferenceReportsArticle/fs/en?CONTENT_ID=4113737andchk=40q4×5 (accessed 07/11/05).

Duncan, E. (2006). Skills and processes in occupational therapy. In: Duncan, E. (ed.) *Foundations for Practice in Occupational Therapy*, 4th edn. Edinburgh; Elsevier, Churchill Livingstone.

Finlay, L. (2004) *The Practice of Psychosocial Occupational Therapy*, 3rd edn. Cheltenham: Nelson Thornes.

Fisher, A. (1997) *Assessment of Motor and Process Skills.* Fort Collins: Three Star Press.

Folstein, M.G., Folstein, S.E. and McHugh, P.R. (1975) Mini-mental state: A practical method of grading the cognitive state of patients for the clinician. *Journal of Psychiatric Research.* **12**: 189–98.

Goldsmith, M. (2002) *Hearing the Voice of People with Dementia; Opportunities and Obstacles.* London: Jessica Kingsley Publishers.

Green, S. and Cooper, B.A. (2000). Occupation as a quality of life constituent: A nursing home perspective. *British Journal of Occupational Therapy.* **63**: 17–23.

Greenberg, S., Motenko, A.K. and Roesch, C. (1999) Friendship across the life cycle: a support group for older women. *Journal of Gerontological Social Work.* **32**: 7–24.

Hedelin, B. and Strandmark, M. (2001). The meaning of mental health from elderly womens' perspectives: A basis for health promotion. *Perspectives in Psychiatric Care.* **37**: 7–14.

Innes, A. (2002) The social and political contest of formal dementia care provision. *Ageing and Society.* **22**: 482–99.

Keilhofner, G. (2002) Gathering client information. In: Keilhofner, G. (ed.) *Model of Human Occupation: Theory and Application*, 3rd edn. Baltimore: Lippincott Williams and Wilkins.

Kitwood, T. (1997) *Dementia Reconsidered; The Person Comes First.* Buckingham: Open University Press.

Kitwood, T. and Bredin, K. (1992) A new approach to the evaluation of dementia care. *Journal of Advanced Health and Nursing Care.* **1**: 41–60.

Lansdown, R. (1994) Living longer? qualitative survival. Meeting report. *Journal of the Royal Society of Medicine.* **87**: 636.

Law, M., Cooper, B., Strong, S., Steward, D., Rigby, P. and Letts, L. (1996). The person-environment-occupation model: a transactive approach to occupational performance. *Canadian Journal of Occupational Therapy.* **63**: 9–23.

Menec, V.H. (2003). The relation between everyday activity and successful ageing: A 6 year longitudinal study. *Journal of Gerontological and Scientific Social Science.* **58**: 74–82.

Mullhall, D. (1993) *Functional Performance Profile.* Berkshire; NFER-NELSON.

Murphy, C. (1994) *It Started With a Sea-shell; Life Story Work and People with Dementia.* University of Stirling: Dementia Services Development Centre.

Okum, M.A., Stock, W.A., Haring, M.J. and Witter, R.A. (1984). The social activity/subjective well-being relation: a quantitative synthesis. *Research on Aging.* **6**: 45–65.

Perrin, T. (1997) Occupational need in severe dementia: a descriptive study. *Journal of Advanced Nursing.* **25**: 934–41.

Perrin, T. (2001) Don't despise the fluffy bunny: A reflection from practice. *British Journal of Occupational Therapy.* **64**: 129–34.

Perrin, T. and May, H. (2000) *Well-being in Dementia: An Occupational Approach for Therapists and Carer.* Edinburgh; Churchill Livingstone.

Pitkin, J. (2004) Validation: exploring beyond the person we see. *Journal of Dementia Care.* **12**: 28–9.

Pool, J. (2002) *The Pool Activity Level (PAL) Instrument for Occupational Profiling; A Practical Resource for carers of people with cognitive impairment*, 2nd edn. London; Jessica Kingsley Publishers.

Powell, J. (2000) *Care to Communicate; Helping the Older Person with Dementia.* London: Hawker Publications.

Psychological Assessment Resources Inc. (1998) *Dementia Rating Scale.* Odessa, FL: Psychological Assessment Resources Inc.

Sacco-Peterson, M. and Borell, L. (2004). Struggles for autonomy in self-care: the impact of the physical & socio-cultural environment in a long term care setting. *Scandinavian Journal of Caring Sciences.* **18**: 376–86.

Seymore, L. and Gail, E. (2004) *Literature and Policy Review for the Joint Inquiry into Mental Health and Well-being in Later Life. Age Concern and the Mental Health Foundation.* London: Mentality (www.mentality.org.uk).

Stokes, G. (2002) The environmental setting of dementia. In: Stokes, G. and Goudie, F. (eds) *The Essential Dementia Care Handbook.* Bicester: Speechmark Publishing Ltd.

Volicer, L., Hurley, A.C. and Camberg, L. (2000). A model of psychological well-being in advanced dementia. In: Alber, S.M. and Logsdon, R.G. (eds) *Assessing Quality of Life in Alzheimer's Disease.* New York: Springer Publishing Company Inc.

Wood, B., Spector, A., Jones, C., Orrell, M. and Davies, S. (2005) Reminiscence for dementia. *The Cochrane Database of Systematic Reviews. Issue 2.* Chichester: John Wiley and Sons.

Zigmund, A.S. and Snaith, R.P. (1994) *The Hospital Anxiety and Depression Scale.* Windsor: NFER-NELSON.

9: Exploring lived experiences of occupational therapy and dementia

Sue Bower

In this chapter I will explore the experience of living with dementia from the perspective of one person, Alice O'Connell. In keeping with the work of Creek (2003), I am not attempting to simplify the lived experience of being an occupational therapist. Nor is there a wish to over-generalise the complex realities of living with a dementia, instead I hope to share with you my understandings of some of the ways we could be an occupational therapist with Alice.

The structure of the chapter is loosely based on the occupational therapy process. I will review of some of the theories that underpin occupational therapy practice with people living with dementia, and go on to explore the use of reasoning and reflexive practice as strategies for exploring our underlying values and power relationships. Subjectivity, uncertainty and complexity are not avoided. They are celebrated and valued.

Objectives

After reading and reflecting on this chapter you should be able to:

- describe and explore different understandings of dementia;
- identify differences between the 'old culture' and 'new culture' of dementia care;
- describe some ways in which occupational therapists may work with people living with dementia;
- describe how you would feel about working with Alice.

Some statistics to consider

- There are nearly 18 million people with dementia in the world.
- At present 66% of people with dementia live in 'developing' countries. By 2025 this will rise to 75%. It is estimated that the fastest growth will be in China, South East Asia, Latin America and the Caribbean.

- In the UK, 1 in 20 people over the age of 65 and 1 in 5 over the age of 80 are living with dementia.
- In the UK, one-third of people living with dementia live alone.
- In the UK, over 18 000 people under the age of 65 are living with dementia.
- The most common form of dementia is Alzheimer's disease (approximately half).

(Source: Alzheimer's Society UK and Alzheimer's Disease International 2005).

A story about Alice O'Connell

Alice is an 80-year-old woman. After leaving school, Alice worked as a farm labourer and during the war she worked as a welder. At 18 she married, and a year later she had a daughter. For most of her life, Alice has enjoyed dancing, and picking up bargains at local jumble sales and charity shops. She also enjoys watching her favourite soaps on TV and going to the local pub.

Alice has lived alone since her husband died 20 years ago. She has one daughter (Ellen), two grandchildren and five great grandchildren, whom she enjoys seeing at least once a week. Shortly after her husband's death, Alice moved from their family home to a smaller house to be closer to her daughter.

Recently Ellen went to see their general practitioner (GP), and told him that she was worried about her mother. She explained how, over the past six months, her mother has had increasing difficulties remembering things. Alice regularly loses house keys, forgets the names of grandchildren, loses large amounts of money, and is not paying bills. For the past three months Alice has not been upstairs, and she eats, sits and sleeps on a small sofa. Apart from going to the local shops, she rarely goes out of the house. Alice has been 'hoarding' food and household items, and Ellen expressed concern to the GP about the amount of out-of-date and rotten food around the house. She was also worried that her mother has recently been putting papers into the gas fire flames as though it was an open fire.

Ellen suspects that Alice is not eating or drinking regularly, and that she has not had a wash or changed her clothes for weeks. When she talks with her mother, Alice insists that everything is okay. Last month Ellen arranged for Alice's gas to be cut off, and decided they needed to go to the GP for help and advice. Alice has no known history of mental health difficulties.

Reason for referral to occupational therapy

The GP referred Alice to the local psychiatrist. Alice attended her out-patient appointment with Ellen. The psychiatrist diagnosed Alice as 'suffering from Alzheimer's disease'. The psychiatrist then referred Alice to the local community mental health team for further assessment.

Additional information, based on an initial visit by two members of the community mental health team

Alice appears articulate, orientated and welcoming. She insists that she does not want or need any help. However, Alice's clothes and skin are dirty and she smells of urine. The house is full of rotten and out-of-date food, and the house is infested with mice and lice. It is not possible to access the kitchen, bathroom or toilet without climbing over bin bags full of rubbish. The kitchen sink is blocked and inaccessible.

Task box 1: Thinking about Alice's story

Take some time to think about Alice, her family and her situation. Try to imagine telling this story from four different perspectives:

- Alice's story
- Ellen's story
- The GP's story
- Your story

How and why may these stories be different or overlap?

Alice's story: whose version counts?

There will be different understandings of the 'reality' of Alice's life BUT who will be seen as the 'expert'? Whose version of the story counts when decisions are being made? This will depend on the power relationships between those involved. Who is disempowered in this case study? Who is relatively powerful? Post modernist theorists, such as Foucault (1980), explore power relations, in particular the links between power and knowledge. Foucault represents power as being maintained by 'discursive practices', such as professional training, academic journals, and conversations. Through these practices, the 'reality' of dementia and of being old is *created* and maintained, for example in lectures, in this book and in case supervision. Rather than empower Alice, our 'professional' discourse is understood as an attempt to accustom her to *our* understandings. The dominant 'professional'/'scientific'/'evidence-based' understandings of ageing and dementia *construct* knowledge. This knowledge then masquerades as *the* 'truth'/'reality' in government policy and thus pervades our practice. This *constructed knowledge* marginalises Alice's lived experiences (e.g. her economic, social and cultural life) and makes assumptions based on understandings of general factors (e.g. what it is to be an old woman with Alzheimer's disease). Post-modernists attempt to expose and challenge the assumptions of 'Western' philosophy and science. They reject the generalised *grand/meta-narratives* (e.g. psychiatry, psychology, and occupational therapy theory) in favour of Alice's version of her story (her *micro-narrative*). Analysing and 'deconstructing' narratives and power relationships can inform how we work with Alice. If you are interested in finding out more, try reading:

- Adams, T. (1998) The discursive construction of dementia care: implications for mental health nursing. *Journal of Advanced Nursing.* **28**: 614–21.
- Bryden, C. (2005) *Dancing with Dementia. My Story of Living Positively with Dementia.* London: Jessica Kingsley.
- Cayton, H. (2004) Telling stories. *Dementia.* **3**: 9–17.
- Clarke, C. (2000) Risk: constructing care and care environments in dementia. *Health, Risk & Society.* **2**: 83–93.

- Clouston, T. (2003) Narrative methods: talk, listening and representation. *British Journal of Occupational Therapy.* **66**: 136–42.
- Finlay, L. (2004) From 'Gibbering Idiot' to 'Iceman', Kenny's Story: a critical analysis of an occupational narrative. *British Journal of Occupational Therapy.* **67**: 474–80.
- Proctor, G. (2001) Listening to older women with dementia: relationships, voices and power. *Disability and Society.* **16**: 361–75.
- Sterin, G.J. (2002) Essay on a word. A lived experience of Alzheimer's disease. *Dementia* **1**: 7–1.

Being an occupational therapist with Alice

In the complex and lived realities of Alice's life and our work as occupational therapists, there are many uncertainties and possibilities. When we imagine being an occupational therapist with Alice, it is important that we are able to:

- describe what we think we would do when working with Alice;
- describe how we would do this;
- justify our practice;
- provide a clear account of why we would work with Alice in this way.

Clinical reasoning and making decisions. When considering the what, how and why of being an occupational therapist with Alice, we need to make decisions. Factors that may influence decision-making include:

- strategies that you use to help you make decisions (e.g. narrative reasoning);
- previous experiences and current skills;
- theory and literature, e.g. understandings of culture, dementia and ageing;
- available evidence for 'good practice';
- values and professional codes underpinning your practice – personal and professional;
- contemporary government/social policy, legislation, local guidance/procedures, and policy directives;
- roles and dynamics in the multi-disciplinary and professional (occupational therapy) team;
- guidance and supervision.

Are there other things that may influence how you will be with Alice? When you ask yourself, or are asked by others, why you would work in a particular way with Alice, it may help to use this list to guide your response.

Literature and theoretical understandings of old age and dementia influence ways in which we may understand Alice (see Task box 2). Such understandings would inevitably influence the ways in which an occupational therapist would work with Alice. In 1997 Kitwood (p. 144) wrote:

'Above all else, the reconsideration of dementia invites us to a fresh understanding of what it is to be a person. The prevailing emphasis on individuality and autonomy is radically called into question, and our true interdependence comes to light.'

In keeping with Kitwood, Perrin and May (2000) argue that as occupational therapists we should rethink the professional prioritisation of 'independence' and instead prioritise the *well-being* of people living with a dementia. More recently this emphasis has been supported by the Audit Commission (2004) report, which encourages us to broaden our understanding of 'healthy old age' to include notions of *interdependence* and *subjective experiences of well-being.*

Task box 2: Understandings of dementia

What are your understandings of dementia? What is this understanding based on? How may your understanding of dementia influence how you would be an occupational therapist with Alice? Below is a summary of the most prevalent theoretical understandings of dementia:

Biomedical and neurological

- Dominates 'Western' understandings of dementia.
- 'Dementia' is used as umbrella term to describe symptoms that occur when brain is affected by a disease e.g. Alzheimer's disease.
- Dementia is understood as having stages due to a progressive disease/neurological damage.
- Main symptoms include: memory loss, changes in mood and behaviour, communication difficulties and perceptual difficulties.
- 'Self' is understood as damaged and eventually lost.

Cultural and person-centred

- Anthropological studies are critical of the marginalisation of non-'Western' understandings of dementia in the biomedical/neurological models (Cohen 1998).
- Influenced by the work of Rogers (1961), Tom Kitwood developed biomedical/neurological models of dementia into a more complex understanding of the experience of living with a dementia (Kitwood 1997). The Bradford Dementia Group continues to develop person-centred understandings of dementia and dementia care (Brooker 2004).
- Self is understood as damaged through interaction with others (*not* lost).
- Dementia understood as a disability.
- Dementia understood as the influence and complex interaction of: neurological damage; spiritual well-being; physical and emotional health; physical and psychological environment; coping strategies; life experiences; cultural context; social interactions/isolation/exclusions.

Developing your understandings of dementia

You can find out more about understandings of dementia by accessing these resources:

- www.alzheimers.org.uk – Alzheimer's Society (UK).
- www.alzscot.org/ – Alzheimer Scotland.
- www.dementia.ie – Dementia Services Information & Development Centre (Ireland).
- Bryden, C. (2005) *Dancing with Dementia. My Story of Living Positively with Dementia.* London: Jessica Kingsley.
- Cheston, R. and Bender, M. (1999) *Understanding Dementia. The Man with Worried Eyes.* London: Jessica Kingsley.
- Kitwood, T. (1997) *Dementia Reconsidered.* Buckingham: Open University Press.
- Parker, J. and Penhale, B. (1998) *Forgotten People: Positive Approaches to Dementia Care.* Aldershot: Ashgate.

■ Perrin, T. and May, H. (2000) *Wellbeing in Dementia. An Approach for Therapists and Carers.* London: Churchill Livingstone.
■ Sabat, S.R. (2001) *The Experience of Alzheimer's disease; Life Through a Tangled Web.* Oxford. Blackwell Publishers.
■ Stokes, G. and Goudie, F. (eds) (2002) *The Essentials. Dementia Care Handbook.* Oxon: Winslow/Speechmark.

Contemporary legislation, policy and guidelines. How may these underpin the possibilities of being an occupational therapist with Alice? Task box 3 provides a list of government policy and guidelines that will have some impact on an occupational therapist working in England with Alice today. The policies and procedures of the community mental health team working with Alice will be based on local interpretations of such national policies and guidance.

Task box 3: Considering relevant policies and guidelines

■ Audit Commission (2000) *Forget Me Not: Mental Health Services for Older People.* London: Audit Commission.
■ Audit Commission (2002) *Forget Me Not 2002: Developing Mental Health Services for Older People in England.* London: Audit Commission.
■ Audit Commission (2004) *Older People – Independence and well-being. The Challenge for Public Services.* London: Audit Commission.
■ College of Occupational Therapy (2003) *National Service Framework for Older People.* London: BAOT/COT briefing. COT (Available through COT website).
■ DoH (1999) *National Service Framework for Mental Health.* London: The Stationery Office.
■ DoH (2001) *National Service Framework for Older People.* London: The Stationery Office.
■ DoH (2005) *Mental Capacity Act.* London: The Stationery Office.
■ Philp, I. and Appleby, L. (2005) *Securing Better Mental Health for Older Adults.* London: The Stationery Office.
■ Sainsbury Centre for Mental Health (2001) *The Capable Practitioner. A Framework and List of Practitioner Capabilities Required to Implement the National Service Framework for Mental Health.* London: Sainsbury Centre for Mental Health.
■ Sainsbury Centre for Mental Health (2004) *The Ten Essential Shared Capabilities. A Framework for the Whole of the Mental Health Workforce.* London: Sainsbury Centre for Mental Health.

Related websites

■ www.audit-commission.gov.uk/ – Audit Commission.
■ www.dh.gov.uk/Home/fs/en – Department of Health.
■ www.dca.gov.uk/menincap/legis.htm – Mental Capacity Legislation.
■ www.scmh.org.uk/ – Sainsbury Centre for Mental Health.

Some reflections on government policy

Policy and the practice that it influences do not operate in a vacuum. The values that underlie policy influence stated priorities, for example the priorities in the national service frameworks.

Since the 1970s successive governments have been increasingly concerned with how to 'square the welfare circle'. The Margaret Thatcher government's ideology was a shift away from the collectivism of the comprehensive welfare state, to a belief in individualism and market forces.

The welfare state and older people have been increasingly viewed as a drain on public resources. The marketplace has been promoted as *the* way of pushing down costs and increasing consumer choice – a notion that remains popular today. In the government's attempts to ration and use welfare resources effectively and efficiently, older people are an obvious target. Ageing has been redefined as an expensive medical condition, and resisting the ageing process is promoted as a social duty.

The growth in the number and proportion of older people, and the relationship of this to increased demands on welfare provisions, is a major demographic consideration. Such concerns are used to justify the judgement of older people living with dementia as an economic burden.

- How do you feel about how the welfare state supports older people living with a dementia in the UK?
- How may government policy influence your priorities in your work with Alice?
- How do you feel the government should prioritise resources in health and social care?

For further reading relating to politics in occupational therapy read:

- Age Concern England. *Policy Unit. Policy Position and Policy Response Papers*. Available online from: www.ageconcern.org.uk/.
- Kronenberg, F., Algado, S.S. and Pollard, N. (eds) (2005) *Occupational Therapy Without Borders. Learning from the Spirit of Survivors*. London: Elsevier Churchill Livingstone, (in particular Chapters 6 and 7).
- Pollard, N., Alsop, A. and Kronenberg, F. (2005) Reconceptualising occupational therapy. *British Journal of Occupational Therapy*. **68**: 524–26.

Based on contemporary policy, theory, and professional codes of practice, occupational therapists can justify a person centred approach to their practice. If we strive to be person centred when working with Alice, this will influence all aspects of our practice. In attempting to be person centred, there are implications for the whole of the occupational therapy process. Before we continue to explore how we could be an occupational therapist with Alice, please take some time to think about another person living with a dementia, Christine Bryden. In 1995 Christine Bryden was diagnosed with dementia, and ten years later she wrote about her experiences:

*'How you relate to us has a big impact on the course of the disease. You can restore our personhood, and give us sense of being needed and valued. There is a Zulu saying that is very true: "**A person is a person through others**". Give us reassurance, hugs, support, a meaning in life. Value us for what we can still do and be, and make sure we retain social networks. It is very hard for us to be who we once were, so let us be who we are now and realise the effort we are making to function.'* (Bryden 2005, p. 127, original emphasis).

Could this be how Alice feels?

Task box 4: Different cultures in dementia care

Based on person-centred understandings of dementia, Kitwood (1997) argued that, as practitioners, we should shift our focus from cognitive deficits and remedial treatment to a focus on the emotional reality of living with a dementia. Changes in understandings of dementia, and resultant changes in the priorities of dementia care, became known as the 'new culture' of dementia care (Kitwood and Benson 1995). The 'old culture' prioritises 'organic' neurological and cognitive changes, and practice has a focus on technical aspects that attempt to measure/slow down/stop/prevent these changes. In contrast, the 'new culture' is based on a humanistic, person-centred approach that strives to enhance the well-being of people living with dementia, and to improve the quality of practice and care provision for people living with dementia.

The 'old culture' views the 'challenging' behaviour of people living with dementia as symptoms/meaningless/in need of control or management. The 'new culture' perceives challenging behaviour as attempts to communicate. This approach aims to enhance well-being by attempting to understand behaviour and to improve the quality of care and practice. The 'new culture' validates the subjective experience of dementia. What is it like for Alice to live with a dementia? Focus is on the whole person, not just impairment/symptoms. Each person is unique, with past, present and future – so much more than the disease label of 'demented'. Just as we are all so much more than any of the labels that are given to us. Changing from the 'old culture' to the 'new culture' of dementia care requires a high level of training and skills, and implies a change in attitude. If you are interested in finding out more, try reading:

- Benson, S. (ed.) (2000) *Person-Centred care: Creative Approaches to Individualised Care for People with Dementia*. London: Hawker.
- Brooker, D. (2004) What is person-centred care for people with dementia? *Reviews in Clinical Gerontology*. **13**: 215–22.
- Kitwood, T. and Benson, S. (1995) (eds) *The New Culture of Dementia Care*. London: Hawker Publications.
- Morton, I. and Bleathman, C. (1988) Does it matter whether it's Tuesday or Friday? *Nursing Times*. **84**: 25–7.
- Parker, J. (2001) Interrogating person-centred dementia care in social work in social care practice. *Journal of Social Work*. **1**: 329–45.
- Perrin, T. and May, H. (2000) *Wellbeing in Dementia. An Approach for Therapists and Carers*. London: Churchill Livingstone (in particular chapters 1, 2, 6 and 7).
- Sheard, D. (2004) Person-centred care: the emperor's new clothes? *Journal of Dementia Care*. March/April: 22–5.

Assessing Alice

Thus, in striving to undertake high quality assessments with Alice we must consider so much more than the 'tool'. How are we to 'be' with Alice? How do our values and skills influence our choice of approach, methods, tools and priorities? Rather than viewing assessments as a stage or tool within the occupational therapist process, it can be more meaningful to understand assessment as interactive and on-going 'running through' the occupational therapy process.

Thinking about good quality assessments

Occupational therapists aspire to a 'holistic' approach; our assessments focus not just on the person, but also on their social, physical and cultural environment. It is increasingly argued that our assessments should also include the political environment (Kronenberg *et al.* 2005). What would be the focus of your assessments with Alice? Possibilities include:

- Engagement and inclusion
- Well-being
- Communication skills
- Occupational 'performance'
- Risk
- Cognitive capacity
- Subjective experience
- Carer experience
- Something else?

Task Box 5: Thinking about assessment

How might you assess Alice? How would you be when you assess Alice? What are the key skills you would need to carry out meaningful assessments with Alice?

Try to justify all your answers. You could use the list on page 165 to help with your reasoning.

Some examples and possibilities

In order to place assessment in context I have chosen to focus on four inter-related areas: engagement and inclusion, well-being, occupational performance and risk. Examples of ways in which this focus can be justified include current literature and theory relating to dementia care (see Task box 2), narrative theory and Alice's story (see Task box 1), current policy guidelines (see Task box 3) and the roles and dynamics of the multi-disciplinary team.

Engagement and inclusion

From the story about Alice we are told: 'For most of her life, Alice has enjoyed dancing, and picking up bargains at local jumble sales and charity shops. She also enjoys watching her favourite soaps on TV and going to the local pub. Alice has lived alone since her husband died 20 years ago. For the past three months Alice has not been upstairs, and she eats, sits and sleeps on a small sofa. Apart from going to the local shops, she rarely goes out of the house'.

Based on contemporary recommendation for good practice (see Task box 4) one aim of working with Alice may be to maintain her personhood. Much of occupational therapy theory documents a positive correlation between meaningful occupation, health and well-being (Wilcock *et al.* 1998, Perrin and May 2000, Kronenberg *et al.* 2005). There is also much written about the need for attachments, relationships, and inclusion in maintaining personhood (see Kitwood 1997, Wey 2000, Whiteford 2000, Parker 2001, Bryden 2005, Yip 2005). Talking about her experiences of living with a dementia, Bryden (2005, p. 127) states:

> *'Value us for what we can still do and be, and make sure we retain social networks. It is very hard for us to be who we once were, so let us be who we are now and realise the effort we are making to function.'*

Well-being

Kitwood (1997) argued that well-being for people with dementia is a direct result of the quality of interactions and relationships. Contemporary literature, theory and policy guidance would justify a focus on Alice's subjective experiences of well-being and interdependence, rather than the more traditional 'Western' occupational therapy prioritization of striving for independence.

Occupational 'performance'

Most occupational therapy theory texts would support a focus on occupational performance with Alice. This focus is at the core of what many occupational therapists understand to be their professional 'specialist' role within multidisciplinary teams. From the story about Alice we are told: 'Ellen suspects that Alice is not eating or drinking regularly, and that she hasn't had a wash or changed her clothes for weeks. Alice appears articulate, orientated and welcoming. She insists that she does not want or need any help. However, Alice's clothes and skin are dirty and she smells of urine. The house is full of rotten and out-of-date food, and the house is infested with mice and lice. It is not possible to access the kitchen, bathroom or toilet without climbing over bin bags full of rubbish. The kitchen sink is blocked and inaccessible'.

From this account, it appears that Alice is experiencing difficulties in some aspects of her occupational performance, such as eating, drinking, washing herself and her clothes, and cleaning her home. We have also been informed that Ellen is worried about these changes in her mother's behaviour. However, there is also an indication that she retains important inter-personal and communication skills. In attempting to assess occupational performance with Alice, we would be trying to find out more about these apparent strengths and difficulties. Such assessments would necessitate an exploration of psychological, cognitive, bodily/physical, social and environmental components that may be enabling or presenting barriers to Alice's occupation. In keeping with a person-centred approach to working with Alice, these assessments could only be meaningful if we explore with Alice her thoughts and feelings about her occupational performance. For example: Does Alice think that she has changed and, if so, in what ways and why? How does Alice feel about the changes? How does Alice feel about not being able to get to her toilet without climbing over rubbish? Would she like to change this?

In addition, it is important that Ellen is included in the assessments, while acknowledging that this will bring different experiences, feelings and understandings to the assessments. For example: How does Ellen feel about changes she has made in her life in trying to respond to her mother?

Risk

Risk assessment and management are integral parts of professional processes within the health and social care practice. Legislation and policies have been produced to guide practice (see Counsel and Care 2001, 2002, and Alzheimer's Society 2003, for practice-based examples). The procedures followed in mental health teams are based on local interpretations of legislation and policy guidance. Occupational therapists undertaking assessments of occupational performance with people living with a dementia often focus on identifying potentially hazardous occupations, for example cooking, personal hygiene, heating and operating appliances (Thom and Blair 1998). From the story about Alice you may be able to identify many changes in behaviour/occupations that may be hazardous/risky for Alice, for example using the gas fire, eating and drinking, access around her home, and rarely going out of the house. You may already be constructing your narrative about the probability of Alice or others being harmed if there are no changes in Alice's situation. Remember – this is from your perspective.

However, it is important that your assessment would follow the agreed risk management procedure of your employing organisation. This should involve guidance on the *sharing* of perspectives (Clarke 2000, Hird and Cash 2000, Gilmour *et al.* 2003), in particular, consider sharing perspectives with Alice, Ellen, colleagues in your team, and your clinical/case supervisor. A potential and important dilemma in the risk assessment is that Alice may be seen as someone who is not able to provide valid accounts or make sound judgements. Her perception may not be taken into account:

> *'key concept in risk assessments is whether or not the service user's judgement about their risk taking or dangerousness is to be taken as valid. This is based on the idea that some groups of people do not have the capacity to make such judgements for themselves.'* (Hird and Cash 2000, p. 14).

Would Alice's judgement be 'taken as valid'? Legislation and guidance on 'mental capacity' and consent should be consulted. One of the key principles of the Mental Capacity Act 2005 is the 'presumption of capacity'. This asserts that we should always presume that some one has mental capacity, despite their diagnosis, unless the results of a formal, designated assessment process demonstrate otherwise (Age Concern 2002, Department of Health (DoH) 2005).

How could we undertake assessments, and why?

For the purpose of this chapter, I have chosen to focus on two assessment methods: observation and narrative. An example of key government policy that could influence the focus and method of your assessments with Alice is the Single Assessment Process. Guidance based on this process should help you to share and co-ordinate information with others involved in assessments with Alice. We could justify using observational and narrative assessments by referring to current literature and theory relating to occupational therapy, assessments, and dementia care.

Observation

Attempting to undertake observational assessments with Alice that are outside her usual context and routine could be disorientating for her, wasting opportunities for meaningful and useful observations, and ultimately produce flawed assessment findings with limited use in informing your intervention plan. Perrin and May (2000, p. 133) warn us of the limits of 'contrived' assessments:

> 'the therapist needs to make observations of how the person being assessed engages in day-to-day life in order to reach a deeper understanding of the whole, living, breathing, thinking, active person within his "natural" environment.'

Undertaking observations of Alice at home, as she engages in her everyday life (contextual and naturalistic), can provide a wealth of meaningful information. While being with Alice, your observations would focus on previously identified priorities, for example:

- *Engagement and inclusion*. How does Alice spend her days? Who else is involved in her life? Can you observe any potential barriers to social inclusion; for example does she appear disorientated when she goes out to the shops?
- *Well-being*. What does Alice think and feel about her life? We have been told that Alice insists that everything is okay. Is this the message you get when she engages in her everyday occupations? What about Alice's non-verbal communication – how can this inform you?
- *Occupational performance*. How does Alice get to the toilet? How does she get a drink? Is she able to use her washing machine?
- *Risk*. Can you observe any risks to Alice's physical and emotional well-being? How does she manage potentially hazardous situations?

Narrative (see Task box 1)

Use of narrative methods in assessment provides an opportunity to gather information from the perspective of the 'narrator', for example Alice or Ellen. Using this method, Alice could tell her own story. This does not need to be a fact finding exercise – indeed it may be difficult for Alice to remember some things accurately. However, this method can be useful in enabling you to develop a therapeutic relationship and gain some understanding of who Alice is and what is important to her in life. Clouston (2003) explores how this method can assist our clinical reasoning.

One dilemma you may be confronted with when reflecting on this assessment is the possible tension between promoting independence and well-being at the same time as attempting to reduce risks. Clarke (2000, p. 84) indicates the usefulness of narrative methods in relation to risk assessments:

'practitioners may emphasise the physical domains of risk identification, such as the risk of self harm or the risk of falling. People with dementia, however, may emphasise biographical domains of risk, such as loss of self-identity and family.'

Key skills

These assessments would require competence in particular key skills, for example:

- establishing person centred therapeutic relationships;
- communication and active observational skills;
- validatory skills. Being able to perceive, interpret and validate subjective and different realities. An ability to focus communication on feelings rather than the more usual focus on content (see Bleathman and Morton 1996, Feil 2002, Morton and Bleathman 1988).

Reflexive skills

Interpersonal and analytical skills that enable us to be aware of how we create knowledge in our day-to-day practice. Being self-aware and able to reflect while doing.

Suggested further reading related to occupational therapy assessments with Alice:

- Bryant, W. and McKay, E. (2005) What's cooking? Theory and practice in the kitchen. *British Journal of Occupational Therapy.* **68**: 67–74.
- Mackenzie, A. and Beecraft, S. (2004) The use of psychodynamic observations as a tool for learning and reflective practice when working with older adults. *British Journal of Occupational Therapy.* **67**: 533–9.
- Perrin, T. and May, H. (2000) *Wellbeing in Dementia. An Approach for Therapists and Carers.* London: Churchill Livingstone.
- Pool, J. (2002) *The Pool Activity Level (PAL) Instrument for Occupational Profiling: a Practical Resource for Carers of People with Cognitive Impairment*, 2nd edn. London: Jessica Kingsley.

Occupational therapy interventions with Alice

Planning

As stated earlier in this chapter, high-quality assessments require us to do so much more than select and use a tool. If the assessment is poor quality, there is little point in attempting to plan the occupational therapy intervention. Good quality assessments are ones that provide useful, accurate and meaningful information that will help the therapist, Alice and Ellen to plan occupational therapy interventions.

Prioritising the content of the plan may involve negotiating with Alice, Ellen, other members of the mental health team, and wider networks. The plan will also need to be 'realistic' in terms of resources available. Based on the result of the assessments and the decisions made about priorities, the process of creating an occupational therapy intervention plan can begin. First, the general direction of occupational therapy intervention with Alice (the 'aims' or 'long-term goals') may be considered. Once these are established objectives and occupations that may enable Alice to move towards the long-term goals can be thought through.

Parker and Penhale (1998) warn us that a common mistake at this stage in working with people living with dementia is to make plans that are unrealistic and/or not achievable. You can try to avoid this by ensuring that you have undertaken high quality meaningful assessments and that you create objectives that begin by taking small steps in the desired direction – try not to set Alice up to 'fail'. Remember, when creating plans with Alice, you may organise the plan according to separate long-term goals, but when you are actually working with Alice, you may be working towards more than one goal at a time.

Before exploring how we could create an occupational therapy plan for working with Alice, you may find it useful to refer to the glossary of key terms and consider the relationship between well/ill-being, quality of life and enjoyment. Let us consider what examples of occupational therapy planning with Alice may look like.

NOTE: For ease of communication and to personalise the plan the name of personnel involved could be written here.

Long-term goal 1

Alice will enjoy going out on a regular basis.
  Focus on: Engagement and inclusion, well-being and risk.
  SMART objectives may include:

- After 1 week: Alice will have established a therapeutic relationship with the occupational therapist and enjoyed a meal at a local cafe/food pub with the occupational therapist.
- After 2 weeks: Alice will have enjoyed a visit to the local supermarket and bought items on shopping list with the occupational therapist.
- After 2/3 weeks: Alice will have enjoyed a visit to a local jumble sale with the occupational therapist. She may also buy some new items of clothing.
- After 4 weeks: Alice will have enjoyed a visit to the local community tea dance with the occupational therapist.
- After 5 or 6 weeks: Any thoughts?

Long-term goal 2

Alice will have a wash and wear clean clothes on a regular basis.
  Focus on: Occupational performance, well-being, and risk.

SMART objectives may include:

- After 1 week: Alice will have established a therapeutic relationship with the occupational therapist.
- After 2 weeks: Alice will have discussed and made plans with Ellen and the occupational therapist about how to clear a safe access to the bathroom, a set of drawers and the washing machine.
- After 3 weeks: Alice will have sorted through her clothes – selecting those to be washed and making a list of any new items to be bought, with help from the occupational therapist.
- After 4 weeks: Alice will have washed some clothes, had a strip wash, and put on some clean clothes, with assistance from Ellen and/or the occupational therapist. It is planned that this will coincide with the tea dance (see objective for goal 1 above).
- After 5 or 6 weeks: Any thoughts?

Long-term goal 3

Alice will eat and drink on a regular basis.
   Focus on: Occupational performance, well-being, and risk.
   SMART objectives may include:

- After 1 week: Alice will have begun to establish a therapeutic relationship with the occupational therapist; discussed and made plans with Ellen and the occupational therapist about how to clear a safe access to the kitchen and food storage areas and to a dining table and chair (this may involve referrals to 'outside' agencies, such as environmental health); enjoyed a meal at a local cafe/food pub with the occupational therapist.
- After 2 weeks: Alice will have written a shopping list for food, enjoyed a visit to the local supermarket, and bought the items on list with the occupational therapist; continued to enjoy a meal at a local cafe/food pub with the occupational therapist.
- After 3 weeks: Alice will have had a meal and drinks every day, with support from Ellen, the occupational therapist, and the occupational therapy assistant/home care worker.
- After 5 or 6 weeks: Any thoughts?

Heading towards long-term occupational therapy goals, and planning for discharge

It is important that these plans remain flexible. This work will need to be continually monitored with Alice along side her long-term goals. This may involve on-going observational and narrative reassessments, to ensure Alice is heading in the desired direction. If working with Alice is not 'going to plan', be prepared to adjust your objectives, colleagues and case supervision will help you to manage this process.

After working with Alice for a few weeks you may begin to introduce another person to assist Alice in meeting her long-term goals. Who this person is, and how they are able to work with you, Alice and Ellen, will be dependent on the structure, resources and priorities of your team, local home care support, and the wider community networks. For example, you may gradually introduce an occupational therapy assistant or home care worker to work with Alice and Ellen. You or your manager may then supervise this person, using the occupational therapy plan as a guide. At this stage you may write an occupational therapy report with recommendations for future support and services for Alice and Ellen. This report may contribute to a more comprehensive report from the mental health team. The structure and use of such reports will be determined by the procedures followed by your team, influenced by government policies, for example the 'Single Assessments Process'. This may be the time where the occupational therapist gradually withdraws from working directly with Alice, or you may plan to work with Alice, with a focus on other aspects of her life.

Evaluating occupational therapy with Alice

Why evaluate? How can we know whether we were of any use to Alice or Ellen? Did they benefit from working with an occupational therapist? We have an ethical and professional responsibility not only to ask such questions, but also to reflect and act on any answers. Ways in which evaluation can be useful include helping us to:

- monitor and adjust the occupational therapy plan;
- develop and improve our practice;
- develop and improve the service provided by the team.

When considering the quality of occupational therapy with Alice, take some time to consider possible barriers to working with Alice in a meaningful way. These may include:

- Alice may be reluctant to engage with you – she may not understand or trust your motives.
- You may not be allocated sufficient time to establish a trusting therapeutic relationship with Alice.
- Alice, Ellen and yourself could have very different and conflicting priorities.
- Can you think of other possible barriers?

What are we evaluating? How may we evaluate our work with Alice? I have chosen three examples of evaluations: SMART objectives, quality of life measures, and reflexivity.

SMART objectives

The 'M' indicates that the objectives created should be measurable. If you plan in this way, you can then re-visit your objectives to see if they were achieved.

Repeated observational and narrative assessments enable ongoing evaluations of the occupational therapy plan, and should enable informed adjustments to be made to the objectives, for example: Did Alice enjoy a visit to the local community tea dance with the occupational therapist, after 4 weeks?

Quality of life measures

Your understandings of dementia and occupational therapy will influence your approach to measuring the quality of occupational therapy and quality of life. If outcome assessments are to be person centred, we need to listen to and act on the subjective experiences of Alice and Ellen, for example: What does Alice think about her life? What does she enjoy doing? What would Alice like to change?

If you would like to know more about how people living with a dementia measure their quality of life try reading:

- Cahill, S., Begely, E., Topo, P., Saarikalle, K., Macijauskeine, J., Budraitiene, A., Hagen, I., Holthe, T. and Jones, K. (2004) I know where this is going and I know it won't go back. *Dementia*. **3**: 313–30.
- Fukushima, T., Nagahata, K., Ishibashi, N., Takahashi, Y. and Moriyama, M. (2005) Quality of life from the viewpoint of patients with dementia in Japan: nurturing through an acceptance of dementia by patients, their families and care professionals. *Health and Social Care in the Community*. **13**: 30–7.
- Katsuno, T. (2005) Dementia from the inside: how people with early-stage dementia evaluate their quality of life. *Ageing and Society*. **25**: 197–214.
- Proctor, G. (2001) Listening to older women with dementia: relationships, voices and power. *Disability and Society*. **16**: 361–75.

Reflexivity

This form of evaluation is linked to the notion of complexity and the use of narrative (see Task box 1). Much of health and social care practice literature promotes reflective practice – that is thinking about/reflecting back on our practice, after the event (reflection-on-action). In addition, Mattingly (1991) asserts that 'adaptive thinking whilst doing' is central to occupational therapy practice (being able to think and act 'on our feet'; 'reflection-in-action'). Taylor and White (2000) argue that reflexivity includes both these forms of reflection, but it also pushes us further. If we are to be reflexive when working with Alice, we need to ask questions about the professional assumptions that influence our practice. What assumptions and professional judgements are we making about Alice, her life and her difficulties? This would include an exploration of the power relations when working with Alice, and an analysis of how we understand and use knowledge when working with Alice. Taylor and White argue that reflexivity is essential for good practice in health and social care. As part of the evaluation process, it can help us to make sense of our practice. Reflexivity in practice can be structured through specific professional strategies, such as careful use of supervision and narrative portfolios. If you would like to know more about reflexive practice, try reading:

- Blair, S.E.E. and Robertson, L.J. (2005) Hard complexities–soft complexities: an exploration of philosophical positions related to evidence in occupational therapy. *British Journal of Occupational Therapy.* **68**: 269–76.
- Clouston, T. (2003) Narrative methods: talk, listening and representation. *British Journal of Occupational Therapy.* **66**: 136–42.
- Finlay, L. (2004) From 'Gibbering Idiot' to 'Iceman', Kenny's Story: a critical analysis of an occupational narrative. *British Journal of Occupational Therapy.* **67**: 477–80.
- Taylor, C. and White, S. (2000) *Practising Reflexivity in Health and Welfare. Making Knowledge.* Buckingham: Open University Press.

Using this chapter

An 'evidence base' may help us to make decisions when working with Alice, but what counts as meaningful evidence and why? If we are to work with Alice, we need to be able to practice both the art and the science of occupational therapy.

As I stated at the beginning of this chapter, I have not attempted to simplify the lived experience of being an occupational therapist. I have also tried not to over-generalise the complex realities of living with a dementia. In doing this, I have not created complex world; I have merely acknowledged its existence. I have shared with you my understandings of some of the ways I would think about being an occupational therapist with Alice.

References

Age Concern (2002) *Capacity and Consent.* Policy Position Paper. London: Age Concern.

Alzheimer's Society and Dementia Care Matters (2003) *Building on Strengths: Providing Support, Care Planning and Risk Assessment For People with Dementia.* London: Alzheimer's Society.

Audit Commission (2004) *Older People – Independence and Well-being. The Challenge for Public Services.* London: Audit Commission.

Bleathman, C. and Morton, I. (1996) Validation therapy: a review of its contribution to dementia care. *British Journal of Nursing.* **5**: 866–8.

Brooker, D. (2004) What is person centred care for people with dementia? *Reviews in Clinical Gerontology.* **13**: 215–222.

Bryden, C. (2005) *Dancing with Dementia. My Story of Living Positively with Dementia.* London: Jessica Kingsley.

Clarke, C. (2000) Risk: constructing care and care environments in dementia. *Health, Risk & Society.* **2**: 83–93.

Clouston, T. (2003) Narrative methods: talk, listening and representation. *British Journal of Occupational Therapy.* **66**: 136–42.

Cohen, L. (1998) *No Aging in India. Alzheimer's, the Bad family, and Other Modern Things.* London: University of California Press.

Counsel and Care (2001) *Residents Taking Risks, Minimising the use of restraint–a guide for care homes.* London: Counsel and Care.

Counsel and Care (2002) *Showing Restraint: Challenging the Use of Restraint in Care Homes.* London: Counsel and Care.

Creek, J. (2003) *Occupational Therapy Defined as a Complex Intervention.* London: College of Occupational Therapists.

DoH (2001) *National Service Framework for Older People.* London: The Stationery Office.

DoH (2005) *Mental Capacity Act.* London: The Stationery Office.

Feil, N. (2002) The *Validation Breakthrough.* Baltimore: Health Professions Press.

Foucault, M. (1980) *Power/Knowledge.* New York: Pantheon.

Gilmour, H., Gibson, F. and Campell, J. (2003) Living alone with dementia. *Dementia.* **2**: 403–20.

Hird, M. and Cash, K. (2000) Powerplay. *Openmind.* **101**: 14–15.

Kitwood, T. and Benson, S. (eds) (1995) *The New Culture of Dementia Care.* London: Hawker Publications.

Kitwood, T. (1997) *Dementia Reconsidered.* Buckingham: Open University Press.

Kronenberg, F., Algado, S.S. and Pollard, N. (eds) (2005) *Occupational Therapy without borders. Learning from the Spirit of Survivors.* London: Elsevier Churchill Livingstone.

Mattingly, C. (1991) What is clinical reasoning? *American Journal of Occupational Therapy.* **45**: 979–86.

Morton, I. and Bleathman, C. (1988) Does it matter whether it's Tuesday or Friday? *Nursing Times.* **84**: 25–7.

Parker, J. and Penhale, B. (1998) *Forgotten People: Positive Approaches to Dementia Care.* Aldershot: Ashgate.

Perrin, T. and May, H. (2000) *Wellbeing in Dementia. An Approach for Therapists and Carers.* London: Churchill Livingstone.

Rogers, C. (1961) *On Becoming a Person.* Boston: Houghton Mifflin Company.

Taylor, C. and White, S. (2000) *Practising Reflexivity in Health and Welfare. Making Knowledge.* Buckingham: Open University Press.

Thom, K.M. and Blair, S.E.E. (1998) Risk in dementia – assessment and management: a literature review. *British Journal of Occupational Therapy.* **61**: 441–6.

Wey, S. (2000) Redefining the possible – occupational therapy in the treatment of the person experiencing dementia. In: Burton, L. (ed.) *Occupational Therapy in Dementia Care.* Crick, Northants: Occupational Therapy with Elderly People, pp. 102–17.

Whiteford, G. (2000) Occupational deprivation: global challenge in the new millennium. *British Journal of Occupational Therapy.* **63**: 200–4.

Wilcock, A.A., van der Arend, H., Darling, K., Scholz, J., Siddal, R., Snigg, C. and Stephens, J. (1998) An exploratory study of people's perceptions and experiences of wellbeing. *British Journal of Occupational Therapy.* **61**: 75–81.

Yip, K.S. (2005) A strengths perspective in working with people with Alzheimer's disease. *Dementia.* **4**: 434–41.

Useful web resources

www.ageconcern.org.uk – Age Concern.

www.alzheimers.org.uk – Alzheimer's Society (England).

www.astridguide.org/ASTRID. Assistive technology.

www.audit-commission.gov.uk/ – Audit Commission.

www.brad.ac.uk/acad/health/bdg/ – Bradford Dementia Group, University of Bradford, UK.

www.dh.gov.uk/Home/fs/en – Department of Health. Includes detailed and updated information on government policy, e.g. national service frameworks.

www.makingdecisions.org.uk/ – Making Decisions Alliance: 'wide range of organisations and groups working with people who may, for a range of different reasons, have difficulty in making or communicating decisions'.

www.dca.gov.uk/menincap/legis.htm – Mental Capacity Legislation.

www.mhilli.org/index.html – Mental Health Foundation, specialist pages on 'mental health in later life'.

www.mind.org.uk – MIND National Association for Mental Health UK.

www.nimhe.org.uk/home – National Institute for Mental Health England. Lots of useful links relating to older people and mental health.

www.scie.org.uk/publications/practiceguides/bpg2/index.asp – Social Care Institute for Excellence. Includes 'Best Practice Guide' in assessing mental health needs of older people.

www.timeslips.org/ – 'TIMESLIPS' Creative story telling with people living with a dementia.

Glossary and key terms

Complexity and reflexivity
Complexity theory challenges traditional 'Western' linear scientific theories. Complexity theorists argue that we can not gain meaningful understandings of everyday life (such as living with dementia or working as an occupational therapist) by isolating and investigating separate components. Complexity theory calls on us to challenge assumptions that best quality practice can be obtained by applying 'scientific' evidence: 'in the world of health and welfare practice, the pursued ideal of dependable scientific knowledge may well prove elusive . . . other approaches which foreground understanding rather than explanation and prediction may more fruitfully be explored' (Taylor and White 2000, p. 5).

When thinking about how to be an occupational therapist we need to explore the complex dynamic systems of everyday life: 'We should be proud of the non-linearity and unpredictability of occupational therapy' (Creek *et al.* 2005 p. 284).

This approach promotes reflexivity as a strategy for using knowledge in professional practice. Reflexive practice promotes the exploration of power relations within health and social care. It also invites us to analyse the way knowledge is constructed, interpreted and used in practice.

Related reading: Complexity and reflexive skills in practice
Blair, S.E.E. and Robertson, L.J. (2005) Hard complexities–soft complexities: an exploration of philosophical positions related to evidence in occupational therapy. *British Journal of Occupational Therapy.* **68**: 269–76.

Creek, J. (1997) The truth is no longer out there. *British Journal of Occupational Therapy.* **60**: 50–2.

Creek, J., Illott, I., Cook, S. and Munday, C. (2005) Valuing occupational therapy as a complex intervention. *British Journal of Occupational Therapy.* **68**: 281–4.

Hyde, P. (2004) Fool's gold. Examining the use of gold standards in the production of research evidence. *British Journal of Occupational Therapy.* **67**: 89–94.

Taylor, C. and White, S. (2000) *Practising Reflexivity in Health and Welfare. Making Knowledge.* Buckingham: Open University Press.

Interdependence
A concept more dominant in collectivist 'non-Western' cultures, but recently began to appear in UK policy literature, for example: 'evidence suggests that the

two most important elements of a strategy for successful ageing should be control and interdependence in contrast to the more conventional description of choice and independence as the core public policy goals for people in later life' (Wistow *et al.* 2003, p. 4). 'Interdependence is a central component of older people's well-being; to contribute to the life of the community and for that contribution to be valued and recognised' (Audit Commission 2004, p. 3)

Audit Commission (2004) *Older People – Independence and Well-being. The Challenge for Public Services.* London: Audit Commission.

Wistow, G., Waddington, E. and Godfrey, M. (2003) *Living Well in Later Life: From Prevention to Promotion.* Leeds: Nuffield Institute for Health.

In vitro

In relation to psycho-social practice this term commonly refers to techniques which are organised in an artificial way or setting. For example gradual exposure to source of phobic anxiety in a non natural setting – spiders in tanks as opposed to in person's bath. Exposure can be controlled and graded.

In vivo

In relation to psycho-social practice this term commonly refers to techniques or interventions which are more naturalistic – take place in a more real life setting and are less contrived.

The life span approach

This approach proposes that a person's physical, intellectual, social and emotional abilities change over time and this is affected by the experiences they have.

The cognitive disability model was developed by Claudia Allen, an occupational therapist who suggests that 'a restriction in voluntary motor action originating in the physical and chemical structures of the brain will produce observable limitations in routine task behaviour' (Allen 1985).

Allen, C.K. (1985) *Occupational Therapy for Psychiatric Diseased: Measurement and Management of Cognitive Disabilities.* Boston: Little, Brown.

Non-standardised assessment

Assessments which have not been standardised – commonly referred to as 'home grown'. These assessments can provide valuable information but need to be used with care and interpretation of results avoided. Often they are most useful as *a part* of the assessment process.

Over-identification

Refers to inappropriate feelings on part of the therapist and manifests itself in potentially unhelpful reactions or responses to the client. For example in a case of childhood sexual abuse this may be an expression of anger towards the perpetrator; a sense of powerlessness to help or feeling overwhelmed.

Personhood

A standing or status that is bestowed upon one human being, by others, in the context of relationship and social being. It implies recognition, respect and trust' (Kitwood 1997, p. 8).

The aim of person-centred care is to maintain personhood. Kitwood (1997) argued that personhood is undermined when someone's rights or needs are ignored/not addressed. He promoted 'Positive Person Work' as an approach to help maintain personhood. This work has since been developed by Brooker (2004) (see Chapter 8). The dialectical model of a person-centred approach was proposed by Kitwood (1993) and suggests that a person's dementia is the result of a complex interaction between personality, biography, health, neurological impairment and social psychology.

Brooker, D. (2004) What is person centred care for people with dementia? *Reviews in Clinical Gerontology.* **13**: 215–222.

Kitwood, T. (1993) Discover the person, not the disease. *Journal of Dementia Care.* **1**: 16–17.

Kitwood, T. (1997) *Dementia Reconsidered.* Buckingham: Open University Press.

Quality of life and enjoyment

Definitions of quality of life often include numerous overlapping domains, such as health status, physical environment, social environment, relative economic wealth, autonomy, self-concept, coping strategies, and well-being. Bond (1999) suggests that approaches to assessing quality of life in health and social care fall into three areas: 'normative', 'economic' and 'phenomenological'. 'Normative' approaches are based on the assumption that an increase in levels of disability is automatically reflected in a decrease in quality of life. 'Economic approaches' are used in conjunction with normative approaches. They are used to ration resources, and exclude people from access to services, for example quality adjusted life years (QALYs). The starting point of 'phenomenological' approaches is subjective experiences – this focus/measure is from the perspective of the person living with the mental health problem/disability. Corner (2003) and Veenhoven (2005) explore the relationship between enjoyment/happiness and quality of life. Until recently most measures of the quality of life of people living with dementia have been normative, with a focus on neurological/cognitive deficits or the external environment. Measures focusing on enjoyment, well-being and personhood are less common.

Related reading: quality of life and enjoyment

Bond, J. (1999) Quality of life for people with dementia: approaches to the challenge of measurement. *Ageing and Society.* **19**: 561–79.

Corner, L. (2003) *Assessing Quality of Life from the Perspective of People with Dementia and Their Carers.* Newcastle upon Tyne: Newcastle Centre For Health Service Research, University of Newcastle.

Fukushima, T., Nagahata, K., Ishibasi, N., Takahashi, Y. and Moriyama, M. (2005) Quality of life from the viewpoint of patient with dementia in Japan. *Health and Social Care in the Community.* **13**: 30–7.

Gabriel, Z. and Bowling, A. (2004) Quality of life from the perspective of older people. *Ageing and Society.* **24**: 675–91.

Katsuno, T. (2005) Dementia from the inside: how people with early-stage dementia evaluate their quality of life. *Ageing and Society.* **25**: 675–91.

Kitwood, T. and Bredin, K. (1992) Towards a theory of dementia care: personhood and well-being. *Ageing and Society.* **12**: 269–87.

Smith, A. (2000) Quality of life: a review. *Education and Ageing.* **15**: 419–35.

Veenhoven, R. (2005) Apparent quality of life in nations. How long and happy people live. *Social Indicators Research.* **71**: 61–8.

Single assessment process (SAP)

SAP was introduced in Standard 2 of the *National Service Framework for Older People*: 'NHS and social care services treat older people as individuals and enable them to make choices about their own care. This is achieved through the single assessment process, integrated commissioning arrangements and integrated provision of services' (Department of Health, 2001, p. 23).

Aims of SAP include:

- to promote accurate and person centred assessments;
- to reduce duplication/overlap in practice;
- to reduce emergency admissions and delayed discharges;
- to promote information sharing across health and social care;
- to ensure that the depth and detail of assessment are proportionate to need.

SAP is a single assessment *process* (NOT a single assessment). The process includes four types of assessment: contact, overview, specialist, and comprehensive.

Smart objectives

'SMART' is a useful acronym for setting objectives: Specific, Measurable, Achievable, Relevant and Time limited. Smart objectives are unambiguous (specific) – what is required is clearly understood, there is a measurement included so all concerned know how achievement will be recognised; they are within the person's capacity/resources to achieve but do involve some challenge; they are relevant to the person and their overall aims hence should be negotiated; and finally they are placed within a time frame which is also achievable.

Standardised assessment

Commonly refers to assessment tools which have been tested for reliability and validity, thus ensuring consistency and accuracy of results. Administration and scoring procedures are clearly explained and 'test norms' identified.

Related reading: standardised assessment

Finlay, L. (2004) *The Practice of Occupational Therapy*, 3rd edn. Cheltenham: Nelson-Thornes.

Survivor

This is usually used when abuse has stopped, although effects from it might still be experienced. It can be used by CSA survivors and has positive connotations.

Victim

Usually refers to the time when a person is experiencing actual abuse and may reflect a person's concept of themselves at that time. Later in the recovery process this term might be unhelpful.

Well-being and ill-being

In health and social care, 'well-being' and 'ill-being' are terms used to refer to the physical and psychological aspects of people's experiences. Psychological ill/well-being is understood as comprising of both cognitive and emotional aspects (how we 'think about' and how we 'feel about'). In their influential paper, Kitwood and Bredin (1992) explore the relationship between relative ill/well-being, the care environment, and cognitive skills. They argue that damaging interactions with a person living with dementia can be more detrimental to a person's well-being than their level of cognitive deterioration. Perrin and May (2000) encourage occupational therapists to explore the relationship between occupation, engagement and ill/well-being. They suggest we move away from the more traditional rehabilitative models of occupational therapy, and that we prioritise the well-being of people living with dementia. The Audit Commission (2004) suggests we broaden our understanding of 'healthy old age' beyond notions of dependence, to include notions of interdependence and subjective experiences of well-being. Understandings of well/ill-being are linked to the notion of quality of life.

Audit Commission (2004) *Older People – Independence and Well-being. The Challenge for Public Services.* London: Audit Commission.

Kitwood, T. and Bredin, K. (1992) Towards a theory of dementia care: personhood and well-being. *Ageing and Society.* **12**: 269–87.

Perrin, T. and May, H. (2000) *Wellbeing in Dementia. An Approach for Therapists and Carers.* London: Churchill Livingstone.

Vascular dementia

Vascular dementia is the second commonest cause of dementia accounting for almost 20% of cases. Caused by damage to arteries in the brain. The commonest type is multi-infarct dementia where the brain has been damaged by repeated small strokes. Other causes are high blood pressure and irregular heart rhythms.

Alzheimer Scotland website: www.alzscot.org/ (accessed 29/01/06).

Index